AIDS — THE PROBLEM IN IRELAND

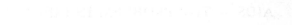

AIDS — THE PROBLEM IN IRELAND

by

Dr Derek Freedman

with contributions by
Dr Zachary Johnson
Fr Paul Lavelle
Dr Raymond Maw

and a foreword by
Dr James Walsh

TOWN HOUSE DUBLIN

First published in 1987 by
Town House
2 Cambridge Villas
Rathmines
Dublin 6

ISBN 0 948524 04 9

Managing Editor: Treasa Coady
Text Editor: Siobhán Parkinson
Designer: Bill Murphy
Printed by: Belfast Litho Printers Ltd.

Contents

This book is dedicated to those infected who have given so generously of time and themselves for medical research, the unsung heroes of this disease, in the hope that we may all learn how to cope, care and contain this infection.

ACKNOWLEDGEMENTS

This book would not have been possible without the help and advice of many people. Treasa Coady, my publisher, whose initiative and enthusiasm for this project, together with gentle and firm cajoling, brought it to fruition. Her editor, Siobhán Parkinson, who put some shape to my English and did not cut too much. Janet McConnell who has kept the whole show on the road and has spent far too many unsocial hours on the word processor, and likewise my secretary, Gráinne Walsh. My colleagues for their forbearance, and my wife and family for tolerating my preoccupation and absences.

I would like to thank Dr James Walsh for his foreword and his encouragement; Dr Raymond Maw, Fr Paul Lavelle and Dr Zachary Johnson for their contributions and enthusiasm and Dr Jonathan Weber of the Chester Beatty Laboratory who read the first draft for me; I very much appreciate his help and suggestions.

FOREWORD

By Dr James Walsh FRCPI, FFCMI

AIDS, or at least infection by the virus that causes AIDS, is by now endemic in this country, though we do not have as many cases as some other European countries. There are already people whom we know to be infected with the virus because they have proved to be positive to the antibody test, and because of this, together with the long incubation period of the disease (seven up to perhaps ten years), it is realistic to say that we are on the edge of an epidemic which will build up over the coming years. The extent of this epidemic will depend on factors in the development of the disease which we as yet do not understand and our capacity to alter our sexual behaviour and intravenous drug abuse.

While one must have faith in the ability of the caring professions to meet the demands which the disease will make upon them together with hope in research providing an answer to AIDS in the form of a vaccine or effective methods of treatment, it has to be said that the prospect of success in either of these fields is not encouraging at this time. This leaves us with the duty of showing compassion to the infected and developing strategies to prevent the spread of infection. Everything possible is being done to protect people from infection by blood transfusion or from blood products (Factor VIII) and there is good reason to believe that these measures are highly effective. The major high-risk areas, sexual promiscuity and intravenous drug abuse, remain as the main challenge if the disease is to be controlled.

It is difficult to anticipate the future pattern of the disease. Is it possible to say how many antibody positive people will go on to full AIDS with its virtually 100 per cent mortality? An optimistic 30-40 per cent or a pessimistic 50-70 per cent? To what extent will AIDS become a mainly heterosexual disease as it is in Africa? What part will neurological AIDS play in the future development of the disease demonstrating the capability of the virus to replicate in the cells of the cerebral cortex?

AIDS is a frightening disease. However, it must be emphasised that as our understanding grows, so it can be contained to a considerable extent by people's own will. People need not be the passive victims of this infection as they are of tuberculosis or other infectious diseases. In confronting AIDS we are masters of our own destiny. However, people must know the facts if unnecessary fears are to be allayed and if the spread of the disease is to be understood and avoided.

There is some evidence to suggest that there is a reasonably high level of knowledge in this country as to how infection with HIV occurs. Unfortunately, knowledge alone may not motivate people, particularly when human sexuality is involved. The problem of the intravenous drug abusers presents its own particular difficulties, which are unlikely to be influenced by media-oriented public health programmes. Given the number of drug-associated cases in Ireland it is essential that this problem receives particular attention.

AIDS is a disease which presents many challenges. One of the most difficult is to provide information in a way that will create the sense of urgency necessary without causing undue panic. The literature suggests that effective information campaigns must distribute the judgements of experts through credible and trusted opinion-leaders, who can effectively channel information to various targeted communities. It is in this context that this book has an important role.

Dr Walsh is Deputy Chief Medical Officer at the Department of Health.

INTRODUCTION

The first inkling I had of AIDS was one morning in July 1981 when I received my copy of *Morbidity and Mortality Weekly Report* from the Center for Disease Control, Atlanta, Georgia. It carried a report of clusters of homosexual men with an unusual form of pneumonia, *Pneumocystis carinii* pneumonia, and a particular type of tumour, Kaposi's sarcoma. I just thought, what relevance does this have for a practising venereologist in Ireland? What will the Americans think of next? How wrong can you be!

That report is interesting in retrospect, as it brought out many of the main features of the AIDS epidemic, as it came to be called, the occurrence of very unusual infections or growths, which had been seen previously only in patients who had an impaired or suppressed cellular immune system (the body's system of defence against disease). The cases occurred in certain groups of people — homosexuals and intravenous drug abusers. It seemed likely that these people were at risk because an infectious agent might be transmitted by blood or sex or through practices associated with their lifestyle. The mortality rate was very high.

In Ireland we remained unaware of the mounting number of cases in the United States, until a review of the AIDS epidemic there was published in September 1982. This caught the attention of the media and the public and a new phase of public awareness began.

One morning I was urgently summoned to sit between a doctor and David Norris on the Gay Byrne Show on RTE radio. The doctor had described AIDS in America the morning before as the gay plague and had associated it strongly with the gay lifestyle, implying that it was the wrath of God. Not surprisingly, David Norris had taken grave exception to this and there had been a heated telephone call to the programme, which aroused a great deal of interest and comment. We knew little about AIDS in those days, except that it appeared in certain risk groups — homosexuals, intravenous drug abusers, Haitians and a few haemophiliacs and recipients of blood transfusions. But we did know that the gay men who had the disease had had a prodigious number of sex partners over their lifetime, 1100 on average in the initial series of cases. It seemed that the condition was possibly associated with the practice of anal sex and use of nitrites or 'poppers' (drugs taken by some homosexuals to increase sexual pleasure). (Subsequently we discovered that anal sex was indeed a high-risk activity, but any connection with nitrites was ruled out.) My scientific and medical background made me feel uneasy about any condition being the wrath of God and I instinctively felt that an infectious agent was a more probable cause. In any case, why should Haitians, haemophiliacs and blood recipients be the subject of the wrath of God? And does God punish those who do not choose their sexual orientation, but find themselves inexorably drawn to a particular lifestyle? Junkies are most probably the product of unscrupulous pushers and social and emotional deprivation, and so do not seem to me to be worthy subjects of the wrath of God either.

To the 218 United States cases reported in 1981 were added a further 790 cases in 1982. By the time I attended the International Society for Sexually Transmitted Diseases Research conference in Seattle in August 1983, the total had increased to 1902 cases. This represented a doubling of reported cases every six months since mid-1981. As well as the Center for Disease Control Taskforce on AIDS, the condition had interested some of the keenest medical and scientific brains in the United States, and began to be the subject of intense study. Most of the studies were centred on volunteer groups of gay men who subjected themselves to regular medical examinations and a battery of tests and procedures, so that doctors and scientists could find out more about the condition. These men could be called the 'unsung heroes of this epidemic'.

At this stage the bones of the epidemic were beginning to be laid out. It was a new syndrome, first described in 1981, but scattered cases could be traced back to the mid-1970s. The number of cases was increasing more and more rapidly, but cases were still confined to certain risk groups — gay men, who constituted the vast majority; intravenous drug abusers; Haitians; haemophiliacs and people who had received blood transfusions; together with a small number outside these risk groups. The epidemic was geographically localised to New York City, San Francisco, Los Angeles and Miami. A small number of cases was reported in Europe, and there were reports of cases in Africa. The African cases and many cases with African links reported in France and Belgium were interesting as they appeared to be heterosexually transmitted. The peak age group was thirty to forty, a decade higher than for other sexually transmitted diseases, which gave an indication of the long incubation period. Case studies clearly showed a sexual or blood link between patients, a pattern similar to hepatitis B. The incidence outside the known risk groups appeared to be very small.

AIDS as a clinical condition was clearly established, and the majority of the patients had either *Pneumocystis carinii* pneumonia or Kaposi's sarcoma (the two conditions mentioned in that first report I had read), although other opportunistic infections (infections that take the opportunity of the body's defences being down to attack it) and other related clinical syndromes began to be recognised, and the 'iceberg phenomenon' was born.

It became increasingly obvious that AIDS only represented the tip of the iceberg — perhaps only 5 to 10 per cent of the people who had the condition. Studies showed that large numbers of gay men were suffering with a type of persistent, generalised glandular swelling known as persistent generalised lymphadenopathy or PGL, but otherwise felt quite well. Many AIDS patients reported this condition prior to the onset of

AIDS, and many of these PGL patients went on to develop AIDS or AIDS related complex (ARC). ARC is where the patient feels quite unwell and has a variety of symptoms, such as weight loss, night sweats, diarrhoea, temperatures, in combination with some laboratory findings that do not make a diagnosis of full AIDS but strongly suggest impairment of the body's cellular immune system. Some people have called this 'lesser AIDS' or 'prodromal AIDS'. A significant proportion of these patients went on to get AIDS. Other clinical presentations were with growths in the glandular system, blood abnormalities, lesions in the nervous system and impairment of brain function to the point of severe memory and concentration loss and dementia.

It was suggested that there was a very large group of people who had whatever caused AIDS, but were completely well and quite unaware that they were at risk of progressing to a lethal illness. This meant that these people could be transmitting whatever caused the condition without realising that they were infected.

Investigations into the mechanics of the condition showed that there was a defect in certain blood cells that constitute the body's defence system or immunity. These are the T-lymphocytes, one of the white blood cells that are responsible for cellular immunity. There was a disturbance in the ratio of T4 lymphocytes to T8 lymphocytes, and the ratio was abnormally low in most AIDS patients. It became known that the disturbance in this ratio was caused by a great reduction in the actual number of the T4 lymphocytes. This was a crucial finding, as this cell is central to the functioning of the entire immune system. Other findings of immune deficiency included a lack of skin reaction to various foreign bodies injected into it, and an impaired immune response to new foreign stimuli.

There were various theories about what caused the condition. It could be a specific infectious agent, which would be blood-borne and sexually transmitted, and viruses seemed a prime candidate. Or it could be an immune paralysis brought about by multiple exposure to various specific antigens, such as agents responsible for sexually transmitted diseases, viruses and foreign proteins as in multiple blood transfusions and injections of Factor VIII in haemophiliacs. The role of nitrites or 'poppers' was explored, and it was also noted that sperm itself was a potent inhibitor of immune functions. Many gays were found to have an abnormal immune function anyway.

During 1982 the first two cases of AIDS were diagnosed in Ireland, and reported in Ireland in 1983. They were both cases of Kaposi's sarcoma in gay men who had had sexual encounters in America and presumably had contracted the condition abroad. In England thirty-one cases were reported by the end of 1983, most of them in metropolitan London and connected with overseas contact.

There was much media coverage on the 'gay plague' and in particular the 'fast lane' gay lifestyle which was common in the areas where most cases of AIDS were seen. There was fear of contracting the condition by casual social contact or by health-care contact, which was fanned by the more sensational elements in the media. There was appreciation that the epidemic would have to be fought by lifestyle changes. San Francisco in particular addressed this issue and became a leader in public health education and in the provision of community care and support facilities, frequently founded by co-operative efforts amongst the at-risk groups.

Almost simultaneously a virus was isolated from patients with AIDS, termed the human T-cell lymphotropic retrovirus (HTLV-III), by Robert Gallo and colleagues in the United States, and from patients with lymphadenopathy syndrome, termed the lymphadenopathy associated virus (LAV), by Luc Montagnier and colleagues in France. These turned out to be the same virus, and that was the end of the speculation over what caused the condition. There was now a direction and an instrument for research to find ways to deal with and prevent the infection.

Isolation of the virus allowed a test to be made for antibodies to it and it became possible to detect who was infected. The iceberg phenomenon was confirmed, with large numbers of people found to be infected as asymptomatic carriers, people carrying the virus — and therefore capable of passing it on — but showing no symptoms themselves. They were mainly in the same risk groups as the AIDS cases, but it became possible to determine the pattern of the infection with a long latent period from the time of acquiring the infection until a clinical condition supervened. A greater variety of conditions was now realised to be associated with the infection and it became clear how the infection had spread into the community before it presented as actual AIDS. Groups such as intravenous drug abusers in Europe, for instance, showed a significant infection rate in certain countries, but there had been only a few cases of AIDS as yet. The risk of transmission amongst sexual partners, men and women, could be detected. The size of the infected population could only be guessed at, but estimates were prodigious — one to one and a half million people estimated in the United States. There was much speculation as to how many of these would progress to AIDS and as to the factors which would be related to this. The development of the antibody test has allowed for screening of blood supplies and has protected the nation's blood supplies from contamination. This, combined with heat treatment, protected haemophiliacs and people who received blood transfusions, and the number of new cases of infection in these groups is now very small.

Hopes for a cure rested on a vaccine, but studies on the virus showed that it changed its antigenic structure quickly, so production of a vaccine would be difficult. Several attempts were also made to find a drug to treat the infection but with little success.

There were six new case reports in Ireland by the end of 1984 but the inexorable rise of cases continued to exceed 5500 reported worldwide by mid-1984. 1985 brought new cases in Ireland and the world total had reached 12,500 by mid-summer. Information and reports of cases flooded in, and the first international conference on AIDS was held in Atlanta, Georgia. It was suggested that the latent period of infection might be as long as fourteen years and the projections for the future were truly horrendous. The value and use of public health education campaigns began to be assessed and issues regarding the use and abuse of the antibody test were addressed.

The media took a spectacular interest in the condition and, while information was given out, a great deal of unnecessary anxiety was induced by highlighting the more sensational and unlikely means of transmission, particularly if it involved a well-known star. The general public began to become apprehensive about the condition and feared infection through ordinary social contact.

1986 brought the total number of cases to over 32,000 worldwide, 28,000 in the United States, 600 in the United Kingdom and fifteen in Ireland. The rate of doubling of the condition in the US had begun to slow down: it was now doubling every ten to eleven months instead of every six months. This was attributed to public health campaigns, counselling centres and general information through the media which has led to a reduction in high-risk activities. Our information about the infection has been further consolidated and the risk of spread into the general community is now recognised.

The infection is taking many more forms, and many common medical conditions are made worse or distorted by the infection. The many guises that the infection can take is reminiscent of syphilis in the days before antibiotics.

The projections for the future are for a minimum of 277,000 cases in the United States by 1991, the vast majority of whom are already infected. These projections, together with the ease of heterosexual transmission and the practical difficulty of changing people's lifestyles for such a basic biological function as the sex drive have brought experts to call this the greatest threat to mankind since smallpox. Reports of large numbers of AIDS cases in parts of Africa, with a significant percentage of the general population infected, cause considerable alarm both for the future of these areas and as a pointer to the way the infection could spread in the western world if measures are not taken to prevent it. 1986 witnessed an unprecedented awareness of the problem by public health authorities and even politicians have devoted funds to fighting AIDS.

At present there is no vaccine, no cure. All we can offer victims is treatment of their symptoms, compassion and comfort, and support from their friends and families. To others we can be more positive: 'Prevention is the only cure — knowledge is the only vaccine.' Public health education should be directed at everybody and people should be ushered into a new era of care and responsibility in relationships. This will also enhance relationships both sexually and emotionally. Perhaps casual sex is an adolescent phase, one which society has just passed through. We are now having to teach our children from the youngest possible age that this aspect of adolescence could be lethal.

We may be sceptical about whether people will change their habits in the face of this lethal epidemic, when they failed to do so for syphilis, which was equally lethal in its time. The difference now is that we are much more open and knowledgeable about sex, we are willing to talk about it and we know the need for direct, explicit information to help people and to prevent them from acquiring the infection.

This is a very sneaky virus. It strikes people without their knowing, often in the middle of men's and women's most pleasurable activities. It lies dormant for many years, but is still infectious by blood and sex. Its presence may not only cause you ill health — it may kill you. You can unwittingly pass it on to your spouse and unborn children with equally lethal consequences. It has the capacity to change society both economically and socially and make us look at ethical questions in a cold objective light, which we have never had to do before. Such is the price of survival. It holds a mirror to society and reveals a soft underbelly that we may prefer to ignore — poverty and exploitation in Africa and among drug abusers, sexual practices we never dreamt of, predictable human weaknesses in most of us and, beneath the surface, the prejudice that fear exploits.

I shall now try to describe fully what we know of the AIDS infection today, how relevant it is to us in Ireland and what are the best practical steps to take to keep it out of your life. I shall attempt to do this at three levels. For the person who wishes to skim through the book, perhaps stimulated by public health and media campaigns, I will try and paint a basic picture of the disease, its manifestations and its effects in Ireland in more detail than is provided in leaflets and booklets. For those who have a particular interest or anxiety I hope I will have provided sufficient detail to answer their questions. And for others who are pursuing projects in this field I hope I can provide a base from which to start.

The book is divided into three sections. Section I is medical, and most readers will probably find the chapter on the virus and the immune system rather heavy going. This chapter is included for the information of people who may be particularly interested in the scientific background to AIDS. The other chapter in section I is on the infection itself, and should be accessible to most people. Section II deals specifically with the situation in Ireland and includes a chapter on the problem among intravenous drug abusers by Fr Paul Lavelle. Also included is a short piece on the situation in Northern Ireland by Dr Raymond Maw. The final section is on advice and counselling and includes a question-and-answer chapter written in conjunction with Dr Zachary Johnson and based on the Eastern Health Board/Gay Byrne Show phone-in. A word of warning — this is a book about a medical topic. Medicine is not a precise discipline and there is much overlap of signs and symptoms between trivial illness and serious illness. It requires the sound judgement of an experienced and knowledgeable doctor to determine what is significant and what is not. A book cannot do this for you.

Section I

CHAPTER 1

THE VIRUS
AND THE IMMUNE SYSTEM

Any real advance in the treatment and prevention of AIDS or HIV infection will depend upon our basic knowledge of the virus, its properties and its interaction with its host and victim. If we are to succeed in conquering the infection, we must know what makes the virus tick. For this reason I am including a chapter on the virus and the immune system, though I am aware that it is not an easy subject. Some readers may prefer to skip this chapter, as it is rather technical, but it is a chapter that you may find yourself coming back to. It carries the ultimate key to conquering this infection.

VIRUSES

The word 'virus' comes from the Latin for slime, stench or poison. Viruses are extremely tiny. Their place in nature is somewhere between living and non-living: their central core is of the genetic materials DNA or RNA and they have the ability to reproduce, but the other structures common to life are absent. They are unable to metabolise, grow or replicate without the help of a host cell. Viruses are the ultimate parasite, models of biological minimalism -- just a core of genetic materials surrounded by a protective envelope of proteins and sometimes fat (lipid).

A virus invades the host cell, usually only one specific type of cell which has cell receptors that interact with the protein on that particular virus envelope. The cell is entered, the virus is stripped of its coat and the genetic material of the virus may pirate or take over the parts of the cell's metabolism involved in making proteins and use up cellular reserves and energy in doing so, either by inserting its DNA (genes) into the DNA of the host cell or as a free gene unit in the cell. Then copies of the viral genetic material are made by replication, and the lipoprotein pattern of the virus envelope is 'translated' through the cell's protein-manufacturing metabolism. The new viral material and the new envelopes come together, and new viruses are assembled, often in large numbers. They are released either by bursting out of the cell, killing it, or by budding out of the cell. The new viral particles then go on to infect other cells in the host or, if transmitted, to infect new hosts.

Some viruses do not go through this cycle of replication all the time. They remain latent or dormant in the cell, some becoming incorporated into the cell's genetic material as a 'provirus'. They await activation by some other agent, a 'co-factor', to begin their replication. The herpes virus is a good example of a latent virus. Once a person is infected the infection lasts for life, even though they do not suffer the symptoms of the illness all the time. For most infections there seems to be a certain amount of viral material required to transfer and establish an infection in a new host — a minimum inoculum.

As parasites, viruses are ultimately dependent upon the survival of their hosts for their own survival. If all the host cells are destroyed, or if the host species becomes extinct, so will the virus. So it is in the virus's own interest, so to speak, to keep the host alive, and the successful virus evolves to live co-operatively with its host, maybe for a very long time and maybe only exerting its effect very subtly over that time. However, even apparently inactive viruses may have long-term consequences, particularly if triggered by other 'co-factors'.

In humans the immune system responds to viral infection and defends the host. Some of the symptoms of acute infections, such as fever, chills, rashes and muscular pains, are due more to the immune response rather than to the virus itself. In most acute infections the body produces antibodies that protect against repeat infections with the same virus. That is why measles is only caught once, and is why vaccination against measles, polio and many other infections is possible.

However, some viruses evade the host's defences by 'changing their coat'. The influenza virus constantly changes the proteins or antigens on its outer membrane, so that antibodies from a previous epidemic are useless: this is why it is possible to catch flu several times in a lifetime, and why injections against flu are only partially successful. Latent viruses even 'hide' by inserting their DNA into the host cell's DNA, where it remains dormant and perfectly concealed from the immune system, but ready to be stimulated into action by co-factors.

RETROVIRUSES

When AIDS came to be investigated, it was thought that the syndrome might be caused by a group of viruses known as the retroviruses.

The retroviruses have a structure like most other viruses: a core of genetic material wrapped in a lipoprotein envelope. However, the genetic core is made of RNA (ribonucleic acid), whereas in other viruses the core is usually made of DNA (deosyribonucleic acid). RNA is the nucleic acid which normally functions in a cell as a messenger carrying genetic code instructions from the DNA of the cell's genes, in the nucleus, to the ribosomes in the cytoplasm, where proteins are manufactured under the instructions of the genetic code.

Each retrovirus particle carries the enzyme 'reverse transcriptase' which copies the RNA of the retrovirus's core into a double-stranded DNA form, the form of the host cell's nucleus. It can then be taken up by the cell nucleus and be inserted into the host cell's DNA. It may remain there forever, hidden from the host's immune system. If the host cell divides, a copy of the viral DNA is passed to each daughter cell. The virus's DNA can pirate the host cell's metabolic machinery to manufacture large quantities of viral RNA, reverse transcriptase and proteins for the envelope. As in the case of the other viruses, the assembled viral particles may be released, either by budding through the cell membrane or, if the virus replicates very rapidly, as in an activated state, by making many viral particles which choke or kill the host cell, which disintegrates, allowing the viral particles to burst out.

Treatment against viruses may be aimed at any of these steps, but the problem is that it may be toxic to the host. Because the reverse transcriptase enzyme is unique in the life cycle of the retrovirus, it is a prime target for antiviral treatment, and many of the agents that have been investigated as possible treatments act against this enzyme.

THE AIDS VIRUS DISCOVERED

A virus was isolated in May 1983 from a patient with a condition known as persistent generalised lymphadenopathy by Luc Montagnier and colleagues from the Pasteur Institute in Paris. Patients with persistent swelling of their lymph glands were known to be in the same risk groups as AIDS patients, many went on to get AIDS and were case contacts of AIDS patients, so it was suggested that the virus that had been found could be the cause, or one of the causes, of AIDS. Researchers had trouble growing the virus, as they found it was toxic to the cells in which it was being cultured.

This problem was overcome when Mikulas Popovic, from Robert Gallo's laboratory in the United States, found a cell culture line of cancerous T-cells that were susceptible to the new virus and were not killed by it. This allowed the culture of large amounts of virus, which gave sufficient material to form a readily available source of antigen for the development of a blood test for antibodies to the virus.

Gallo's group's success was reported in *Science* in May 1984. Accompanying articles described the isolation of the virus from people with AIDS, pre-AIDS, mothers of children with AIDS and one asymptomatic homosexual. It was clear that the virus must be related to AIDS, because when people with no history or connection with the illness and who were in low-risk groups were tested, they did not have antibodies to the virus. The antigen of the virus and antibodies produced against them were analysed and showed that while the new virus was clearly distinguishable from HTLV-I and HTLV-II, two other human retroviruses that had been discovered, it was significantly related to them and was a member of the human T-cell lymphotropic virus family. These groups of findings suggested that HTLV-III, as the new virus was called, might be the primary cause of AIDS, and it was very similar to the virus isolated later in France.

The blood test for the presence of antibodies provided a tool for sero-epidemiological studies and the extent and shape of the 'iceberg' began to emerge. Sexual transmission was demonstrated in case studies. Blood recipients who developed AIDS were able to have the donors identified and the natural history of the disease could be traced as it was transmitted from one person to another. The antibody test virtually eliminated the risk of contracting AIDS through blood transfusion.

The identification of the virus as the cause of AIDS was a landmark discovery which gave direction to the fight against AIDS and allowed realisation of the extent to which this infection had permeated the community. The virus is now called the human immuno-deficiency virus or HIV, and that is how it is referred to in this book.

TRANSMISSION OF THE VIRUS

The virus has been isolated from many body tissues and fluids. As well as the obvious blood and semen, it has also been isolated from saliva, tears, secretions from the cervix and vagina, urine and breast milk. However, it is only known to be transmitted by blood and sex, and is much more difficult to catch than hepatitis B for instance. In studies where a group of health-care workers were exposed to potential infection by both hepatitis B and HIV viruses, only hepatitis B was transmitted and no one was infected with HIV. Consequently, hepatitis B precautions are more than sufficient to prevent transmission of the HIV.

The virus can survive outside the body, particularly in blood products. There is always a time when the viral particles are in free circulation as they transfer from one cell to another. The virus can be maintained in a viable state for several months in a freezer at $-70°C$. It will survive in blood and blood products stored in a fridge and it will survive lyophilisation, a technique used in the preparation of Factor VIII for haemophiliacs. It will even survive for ten days dried out on a glass or plastic dish in a laboratory. It is unlikely, though, that it would survive outside the body in sufficient quantity to establish infection.

It is easily inactivated by the various chemical disinfectants used in medical and dental practice. A low concentration of domestic bleach (Domestos for instance) (1:10 sodium hypochlorite) is adequate for washing floors, clinical areas and dealing with blood spillages.

The virus can be inactivated by boiling or autoclaving (a sterilising process involving steam) and this is the best way of dealing with medical and dental instruments. Heating the lyophilised Factor VIII required for treating haemophiliacs at 68°C for seventy-two hours or the liquid form at 60°C for ten hours will eliminate the virus effectively. This is now done as a routine measure to prevent new transmission of the virus to haemophiliac patients. They are also protected by the routine screening of all blood donors against this infection.

THE VIRUS AND THE IMMUNE SYSTEM

A human being is not only being continually bombarded by new foreign particles, which include infectious agents such as bacteria and viruses, but he or she also has a number of 'silent' infections present which were picked up in early life and have remained contained or damped down by an immune system in good working order. *Pneumocystis carinii* pneumonia may be one such infection, to which a large number of people in the western world are exposed in childhood, and which is dealt with by an intact immune system. However, with breakdown of the immune system, the infection activates and causes pneumonia. Similarly, we are seeing new cases of tuberculosis (TB) in patients who were infected many years previously, where the infection had resolved, but then reactivated in the absence of an intact immune system.

The spectrum of infections seen with AIDS may differ from place to place and from population to population and reflects the past infections latent in each particular group as well as current ones in the community. The immune system probably also acts to keep abnormal cells, like cancerous cells, in check so when the system is defective the cancers can grow and take hold. It is noteworthy, though, that only a certain limited range of infections, the opportunistic infections like *Pneumocystis carinii* pneumonia and certain cancers like Kaposi's sarcoma or B-cell lymphoma are facilitated, and the body seems to retain a defence to many other commonly encountered infections, such as influenza. In other words, even in people with fully developed AIDS, the immune system has not broken down completely.

HIV and the T4 cells
The AIDS virus damages the immune system by attacking the T4 lymphocyte cells. Lymphocytes are white blood cells, and they fall into two main groups: T4 or helper cells and T8 or suppressor cells. The T4 lymphocyte is central to the immune response and has been dubbed 'conductor of the immune orchestra'.

HIV is positively attracted to the T4 lymphocyte cells and interacts with the T4 receptor, possibly to provide entry into the cell. The virus has also been shown to grow in the brain and it is thought that it grows in cells that derive from the same stem cell as the T4 lymphocytes and bear the same receptor.

The hallmark of AIDS is the destruction of T4 lymphocytes and this is the prime deficit in AIDS which causes the loss of immune functions. In AIDS there is both a reduction in the number of T4 lymphocytes and an impairment in their function.

Recognition of particles and agents that are foreign to the body is basic to immunity. The recognition sites are foreign proteins called 'antigens'. Hand in hand with recognition goes specificity of reaction to them, so that only the foreign antigens are sought after and destroyed. There is also memory involved, as the system has the capacity to recognise and react more quickly to previously encountered invaders. This ability to remember is the basis of natural immunity and vaccination.

The monocyte/macrophage series of blood cells are the first ones to react to an invader. They take up the antigen, reduce it and fix it in a form that generates a strong response. It produces a protein, Interleukin I, which activates the growth, development and function of the T4 cell by turning on the genes for a growth factor, Interleukin II, and receptors for Interleukin II on the cell surface. Interleukin II, when bound to the receptor, starts a rapid proliferation of the cells, resulting in a clone of perhaps a thousand descendants, all programmed to respond to the same foreign antigen.

These descendants circulate in the blood and if they encounter the specific antigen for which they are programmed, they activate the 'effector arms' or killer arm of the immune system — the B-lymphocytes and their daughter cells, the plasma cells, which produce antibodies; and the T8 cytotoxic lymphocytes or killer cells which attack the pathogens (invading agents) and the cells they infect directly. The antibodies are specific to the foreign antigens. They coat them, neutralise them, or, if they are part of a larger complex such as a virus or a bacteria, they provide recognition sites for the cytotoxic T8 cells and macrophages.

The T4 cells stimulated by the foreign antigen and Interleukin I are termed activated T-cells. They are in a state of great activity, multiply rapidly and secrete many small proteins which reinforce their activity, replication and expression of relevant genes.

One can see the central role of these activated T-cells for recognition, organisation and destruction of foreign antigens.

THE IMMUNE DEFECT IN AIDS

Initial infection with HIV is met by an immune response and the production of antibodies. This may produce an illness in a small proportion of people: the sero-conversion illness. The response, however, does not succeed in neutralising or killing off the virus. The antibodies are termed 'non-neutralising' antibodies. The virus persists, in a latent or provirus form, in the host target cells — the T4 lymphocytes and macrophages. The potential end result is an absolute reduction in the number of T4 lymphocytes — the hallmark of AIDS. This brings about a reversal of the ratio of T4:T8 cells normally seen in the blood. Not only are the T4 cells reduced quantitatively, but also they are affected qualitatively. They do not function in response to antigens, either by making new antibodies or by inducing T8 cytotoxic killer cell activity. The monocytes also are affected and have a defective response to foreign antigens. Whether this occurs progressively with the passage of time at a constant rate, or is induced by co-factors, is a matter of intense speculation.

Antibody production is affected with a converse effect. Antibody levels are elevated, and all the B-cells are activated, mature and producing antibodies — polyclonal activation. But they are all old antibodies and there is an inability to make new antibodies in response to a new infection or antigen.

The consequence is that an HIV-infected person cannot mount an antibody response to a new infection which reduces the ability to fight and resist new infections. Combined with this there is a defect in the natural killer cells and cellular mediated immune function is reduced. Many of the clinical signs and symptoms that help us to make diagnoses in medicine are dependent upon the immune system producing an inflammatory response to infection mediated by the immune system. These are often blunted in HIV-infected people and AIDS patients, which makes diagnosis more difficult and infection more widespread before it becomes apparent.

HOW THE IMMUNE DEFECT IS BROUGHT ABOUT

If we knew how the immune defect is brought about we would have a much more accurate knowledge of the disease process and a more precise ability to advise infected people. We would also be in a better position to develop treatment for those already infected. Isolation of the virus enabled us to advise people how to avoid infection, and knowledge of the mechanisms of how the immune defect is wrought may lead to a more effective therapy for those already infected.

We need to know what events at the cellular level bring about this clinical catastrophe. The specific target of the virus is the T4 molecule seen on the T4 lymphocytes and monocytes. Activation by a foreign antigen of the infected T4 lymphocyte produces not the clone of nearly a thousand cells seen normally, but a stunted clone with as few as ten cells, which, when stimulated by an antigen, begin to produce viruses and die.

The T4 molecule and the viral envelope protein

The T4 molecule and its interaction with the virus may provide one avenue for explaining what is happening at cellular level. The virus most likely gains entry to the cell by an interaction of the outer envelope of the virus and the T4 receptor. One part of the viral outer envelope, lipoprotein, appears to interact with a T4 molecule and the virus is drawn into the cell by the cell membrane wrapping around it and forming a vesicle, or small bubble inside the cell. Cell death occurs with production of the virus and some evidence associates the T4 molecule with cell death. The rate of cell death may be dependent upon the amount of T4 on the surface membrane. Passage of large numbers of viral particles may produce too many perforations in the cell membrane, allowing vital constituents to leak out, resulting in cell death.

Another possible mechanism involves the envelope protein of the virus. In its interaction with the T4 receptor it straddles the cell membrane, one portion reacts with it and the other is externalised (it sticks out of the infected T4 cell). This externalised portion of the viral envelope lipoprotein may interact with other cells carrying the T4 molecule and the virus and cause them to fuse together forming multinucleated giant cells — syncitia formation. These are many hundreds of cells and because one cell can directly infect another, the potential is there for one infected cell to kill hundreds of others, without their coming into contact with antibodies which may be present in the blood. Even the expression of envelope protein on cells that do not have many T4 molecules, such as a macrophage or follicular dendritic cell in lymph glands, would allow them to interact with T4 cells to form syncitia, mopping up and killing the T4 cells. The importance of this mechanism has still to be determined.

Viral activation

A central question about this infection is how and why the virus changes rapidly from an almost dormant 'provirus' state to a state of high activation with a rate of replication many times higher than that seen with other viruses, high enough to kill the host cell.

Replication, or the manufacture of new viral particles, is controlled by expression of the viral genome which is present in the host cell in its DNA form, integrated into its host DNA as a 'provirus'. Present investigation reveals that the viral genome of HIV is much more complicated than in other retroviruses. A genome can be broken down into its respective parts by cutting it up with enzymes and splicing it together

HIV GENOME

Genes, Gene Products and Function

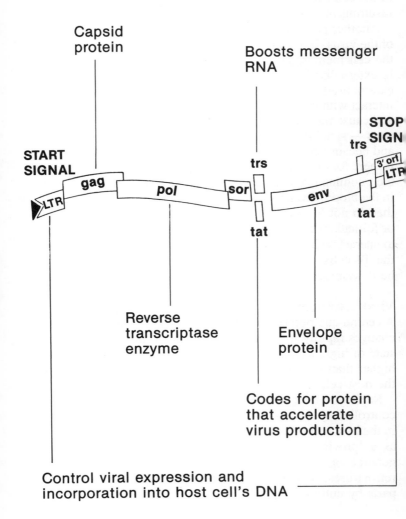

in different forms, sometimes in different host cells to test what each part does. The HIV was found to have the basic genes found in all retroviruses: *ENV* which codes for the envelope protein, *GAG* which codes for core proteins and *POL* which codes for reverse transcriptase. These three genes have sequences called *LTR* (long terminal redundancies) at either end and they include DNA sequences that have a role in controlling the expression of viral genes and are responsible for integrating the DNA provirus copy into the host cell's DNA.

HIV has four extra genes, some of which may be involved in regulating viral expression. They are called *TAT, TRS, SOR* and *3' ORF.* They are present in infected people, as antibodies against them are detectable. *TAT* or transactivator gene, so named because it exerts its influence at a genetic site distant from its location, is present in two reading frames in HIV, in the middle rather than at the end. It encodes for a protein that massively accelerates viral replication in combination with another gene, *TRS*, which is essential for viral replication. *TRS* facilitates the function of messenger RNA which cannot work without it. In other words, *TRS* may act as a kind of 'lock' on viral replication and may be a factor in determining how the virus lies dormant for so long until activated. The recognition that viral replication requires both *TAT* and *TRS* genes together gives a potential target with which to interact a specific agent or drug to block it and it may have some future therapeutic usefulness.

Latency

The great enigma is: what activates the virus from latency to activity? A latent infection where the cell contains the viral genome as a 'provirus' appears to be normal and survives its normal lifespan. The conversion of a latent infection into a productive active one with viral replication can be artificially induced in a cell culture system in a laboratory by the addition of co-factors to latently infected cells. Such co-factors include mutagenic chemicals that cause gene inactivation, foreign antigens and T-cell growth factors, such as Interleukin II. The genetic sequences for coding for HIV activation may be similar to the activating genes of the T-cell. Interleukin II genes and gamma interferon genes have regulatory sequences that have some genetic sequences in common with (and may be mistaken for) the activating sequences of HIV.

It may be that if an infected T4 cell is activated by a foreign antigen, lymphokine genes are expressed to make interleukins and interferon. The activated genes of the provirus may be turned on by the peptides inducing Interleukin II and gamma interferon, which, if *TAT* and *TRS* were involved, would result in very fast replication, leading to the cell becoming a 'virus factory', eventually leading to cell death as the viruses burst their way through the cell membrane and destroy the integrity of the cell. Much of this may be speculation, but if the molecular mechanism for activation of the virus involves small peptides and genetic sequences that are in common to T-cell activation, that would explain why expression of the virus may be linked to activation of T-cells by co-factors such as other infections.

Some correlation has been seen between disease expression and concurrent infections with other sexually transmitted diseases. Short incubation periods are seen in the newborn where the immune system is in a state of higher activation as the immune repertoire is being learnt. A high rate of disease expression is seen in pregnancy, where the presence of the foetus may act as a foreign antigen to an immune system, which is suppressed so as not to reject it. In Africa there is a constant bombardment of the immune system by a multitude of parasites and bacteria. However, there is no proof of special co-factors inducing expression of AIDS in infected individuals, and recent studies have shown that duration of infection is the most important factor in determining the development of AIDS in infected individuals. But of course the longer you have the infection, the greater the chance of exposure to other infections. Identification of specific co-factors would greatly benefit infected people, who would then try to avoid them, and would allow investigation into therapy that would slow down the activating mechanism and reduce the chances of disease progression.

In the meantime it would be prudent to advise infected people to avoid exposure to other infections, particularly sexually transmitted diseases and other chronic infections that would stimulate the T4 activating system. Such advice is easy to give but often hard to live up to.

TREATMENT

Various substances have already been tried to intervene at the T4 receptor, but they have either been ineffective or too toxic for use. The uniqueness of the reverse transcriptase enzyme and the fact that it does not occur in normal human cells allows a target with potential to be efficacious against the virus, yet not be too toxic to the host cell.

Azidothymidome (AZT) is a chemical analogue of one of the DNA nucleotides which the viral reverse transcriptase will incorporate into a growing proviral DNA chain. However, it lacks the correct subunit for the next link in the chain, and the DNA chain cannot continue to be made. The abnormal chain cannot be integrated into the chromosomes as a 'provirus', nor can it replicate, so the spread of infection is halted.

Initial tests with AZT have shown promise. Patients treated showed improved well-being, weight gain and resolution of some of their opportunistic infections. It crosses the blood brain barrier and in a small series of cases some reversal of the defects of HIV encephalopathy was seen. However, it is a toxic drug, and many have had to stop treatment because of bone marrow depression causing anaemia. Its usage will require constant medical supervision at a sophisticated level. It will be very expensive and although at present its use is restricted to AIDS patients subject to special surveillance only, one would wonder what it would cost to treat the millions of people known to be infected. It is not curative, but it appears to slow down or halt the progression of the disease and prolong active life with AIDS. Ultimately however, it has no effect on the inevitable outcome.

Most antiviral drugs show maximum effect if they are used early in the course of a disease. However, a person with AIDS is in the final stages of HIV infection. It will be very exciting to see the results of trials being conducted to find out if it is effective if used early in the course of the infection. It may lead to the development of newer, less toxic and less expensive derivatives.

Viral variation and vaccines

HIV frustrates by its considerable genetic variability, which is expressed as variation in the structure of the envelope protein antigens. HIV has many strains, some varying by as few as eighty nucleotides of the 9500 making up the viral genome, others differ by more than 1000. This variation of the nucleotide which codes for viral proteins is expressed as variations in the viral proteins. These may account for strain differences in the biological activity of HIV, perhaps including preferences for infecting either T4 cells, macrophages or the brain. It is interesting to note that HIV-infected people in the United States show a higher proportion of HIV encephalopathy than their counterparts in Europe.

This variation is shown not only between individuals, but also within an infected individual who may harbour several closely related strains of the virus. Individuals appear to be infected with a 'cluster' of closely related viruses, a group of which seems to dominate at any given time, but the dominant group may change with time.

The fact that they are closely related in their genetic make up may mean that they have the ability to prevent infection with more distantly related strains and that the body has a capacity to mount such a protective immune response.

While there have been developments in the delivery of viral antigens to the body in order to produce a more effective and prolonged immune response, no vaccine as yet has been able to cope with the profusion of different strains. It is similar to the position with the influenza virus. Whilst technically we can make a vaccine for the specific type of virus, we are unable to produce a vaccine that will cover a multitude of strains, some of which are newly appearing.

Perhaps research will guide us to an antigen in the virus that remains constant and may become a target for vaccination. Until then we will have to wait. We also have to be wary. Any 'AIDS vaccine' may be taken by millions of people. HIV infection has a particularly long latent period and time-scale of evolution of its clinical spectrum. It will take some time to show that any vaccine is safe for use and that it will not have any harmful long-term side effects.

CHAPTER 2

THE INFECTION

A person infected with the human immuno-deficiency virus (HIV — the virus that causes AIDS and the other milder conditions associated with it) may be at any stage of infection as shown in the diagram.

The first stage is infection with the virus. The infected person does not know they are *infected*, as there are no signs or symptoms in the early stages, and may not be for several years: the infected person is an *asymptomatic carrier*. If a person suspects they are infected they may have an antibody (HIVab) test done, and if they are indeed infected, they will show up as antibody positive (HIVab+), if the test is carried out at least three months after exposure to the virus, as it takes this long for the antibodies to the virus that the test recognises to be reliably present. An asymptomatic carrier (whether or not they have been tested and shown to be HIVab+) may continue to appear healthy for a long period, perhaps for several years, because the virus lies dormant in the system.

But shortly after contracting the infection, a few patients may develop a *sero-conversion* illness. This happens around the time that the body is producing antibodies to the virus. It is a flu-like illness which may easily go undiagnosed.

The next stage of the infection is either *persistent generalised lymphadenopathy* (PGL) or *AIDS related complex* (ARC). With either of these conditions the patient is more likely to be diagnosed, but PGL can go unnoticed. The person may recover

STAGES OF HIV INFECTION

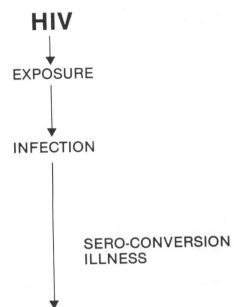

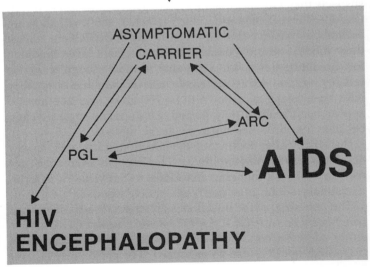

from either of these stages and revert to being an asymptomatic carrier, or may develop one of these stages from the other, or may go from either of these stages to *full AIDS* or to *encephalopathy*, which is caused by the virus itself rather than by an opportunistic infection or tumour.

We are now beginning to see a very wide range of conditions associated with this disease. AIDS itself is diagnosed when a person presents with one of the opportunistic infections that are characteristic of this illness. Some of these, such as *Pneumocystis carinii* pneumonia, are unique to AIDS patients, as in normal, healthy people they do not give rise to any disease. Other infections, such as toxoplasmosis, candidiasis and herpes, do cause mild, localised, short-lived disease in the normal person, but in the immuno-compromised patient they cause a more persistent, severe, and in some cases progressive disease. And then there are organisms that cause significant disease in normal people, but when the patient is immuno-compromised the normal immune reaction does not take place, leading to disseminated infection which may respond poorly to treatment. An example of this is tuberculosis (TB).

The commonest opportunistic tumours are Kaposi's sarcoma and a B-cell lymphoma. These are more aggressive and present in unusual forms in different positions in the body in the immuno-compromised patient. It has been suggested that these tumours may be the result of infection by other viruses, particularly human herpes virusus which have a known cancer producing potential, and that the immuno-deficiency state allows them to become manifest in an aggressive form, but there is no proof of this.

Primary infection with the virus itself (as distinct from opportunistic infections) is thought to account for the effect on the brain, either that of a mild deterioration in intellectual function or a progressive encephalopathy leading to total dementia.

The chances of a person's acquiring the infection depend upon how many people are already infected in the population or subgroup of the population to which you belong, or to which you expose yourself, and how often you expose yourself to the risk of infection by sex or blood.

If you go on to develop AIDS, the actual presenting opportunistic infection or tumour will depend on which organisms are already latent in your own body, as well as the organisms in the environment. Kaposi's sarcoma, one of the first markers of this condition, is now declining in frequency, while HIV encephalopathy is increasing, reflecting a difference in their latent periods. As the number of cases increase, new clinical manifestations are seen: as our knowledge of the infection increases people are altering their lifestyle and consequently having less exposure to the 'co-factors' (factors which trigger off disease in infected people) as well as being in general more health-conscious.

The nature of the virus itself may change with time, as it undergoes continuing variation and mutation. Fortunately the trend in the past for other virus infections has been that they become weaker as they establish themselves in a community, either because the virus itself changes, or maybe because it has 'knocked off' the weaker and more susceptible members of the community first and the remainder are more resistent to infection.

ACQUIRING THE INFECTION
The human immuno-deficiency virus (HIV) has been described as something you have to 'work hard at' to catch. There is no evidence at all of transmission of the virus contagiously, like flu, polio or measles. No one has been able to demonstrate its transmission by ordinary social contact: case studies of cases of AIDS and HIV infection in households have confirmed that it is not passed by sharing eating utensils, toilets, towels , nor even by kissing. Studies in schools with infected haemophiliacs have shown no transmission even in the rough and tumble of the everyday life of youth. In the United States, where cases of AIDS number nearly 30,000 and estimates of numbers infected in the community exceed one million, the unexplained cases of AIDS have remained at around 6 per cent and none of these clusters in any particular population group which one would expect to be exposed frequently to risk of transmission from the high-risk groups. Even with health-care workers who have had a large degree of exposure to potentially infected

material, there have scarcely been a handful of reports of unexplained infection. For every patient there must be more than ten health-care workers with whom they come into daily contact, so the potential numbers exposed to infection would be very large indeed.

There have been a few scattered reports of health-care workers becoming infected by needle-stick injuries. This is where the nurse or attendant stabs themselves with a needle which has been used in an infected person. The first case involved a nurse in England who gave herself a micro-injection of blood by accident, having just taken a sample from an infected patient. She developed a sero-conversion illness some weeks later. Another case involved an orderly who received a deep intramuscular stab by a cannula, a large bore needle, that had been used in an infected patient. Over a thousand simple needle-stick injuries have been followed up and only one has been shown to result in infection. More interestingly, in a study of needle-stick injuries from patients who were infected with both the HIV and hepatitis B virus, infection of the health-care worker with hepatitis B took place readily while no infection with HIV occurred. This suggests that quite a large amount of HIV would be needed for transmission of infection to be likely. So we conclude that this is a virus that is transmitted only by blood and sex, and from mother to foetus.

Blood transfusions

Transmission by blood is easy to understand. In the early stages of our knowledge of this disease, people who received blood transfusions, where the virus was directly transfused from one person to another, became infected. Usually this only happened where the person received multiple units of blood, in much the same way that people with multiple sexual partners are at risk, because naturally a person's chance of becoming infected increases with the number of potential sources of infection to which they are exposed. However, infection also occurred in some cases from one source only. Haemophiliacs were more open to infection because the Factor VIII blood product they received was prepared from a pool of several thousand donors. Today screening of all blood donors for HIV infection means that there are virtually no new cases of infection by blood transfusion. There is of course absolutely no risk of catching this infection by donating blood.

Drug abusers

The virus can be passed between intravenous drug abusers if they share needles, syringes or 'works'. Blood is drawn up into the syringe and mixed with the drug before injection, so there is residual blood left in the end of the syringe and on the needle to be mixed with the next person's blood, and this would be of sufficient volume to transmit the infection. Infection among drug abusers was most common initially in Manhattan, where the carrying of needles and syringes is a criminal offence, so abusers went to 'shooting galleries' where they rented the 'works'. These were often shared by up to one hundred people who also shared the potential of becoming infected. In Scotland a large proportion of intravenous drug abusers in Edinburgh are infected, compared with only a small proportion in Glasgow. This has been attributed to a police clamp-down on the availability of needles and syringes, resulting in much sharing of the 'works'. It is hard to know whether it would be a good thing to make clean needles available to addicts: on the one hand it is not a good idea to encourage drug abuse, but on the other hand, if drug abusers used clean needles then they would not be spreading this disease among themselves and possibly into the community at large, through sexual transmission to non-drug abusers.

Sexual transmission

Penetrative sexual intercourse either homosexual or heterosexual is an efficient transmitter of the infection. In homosexual sex, most cases are associated with passive anal intercourse. Studies show that insertive anal intercourse is less risky, and that oral sex, even where semen is swallowed, is quite low risk. In a recent study from the Multicentre AIDS Cohort Study (MACS) where 2500 homosexual men, who were negative for HIVab, were followed for six months, 3.8 per cent became infected. 10.6 per cent of those who practised receptive anal intercourse with two or more partners became infected over six months, compared with 0.5 per cent of those who did not engage in receptive anal intercourse but had insertive anal intercourse. No HIV infection occurred in those who did not practise either receptive or insertive anal intercourse. Anal intercourse was found to be the only significant risk factor for HIV infection with the risk increasing from three fold for one partner to eighteen fold for five or more partners. Data for the two successive six month periods showed that men who reduced or stopped the practice of receptive anal intercourse significantly lowered their risk of becoming infected to 3.2 per cent and 1.8 per cent respectively. Receptive anal intercourse accounted for nearly all new HIV infections amongst the homosexual men enrolled into the study. It is of particular note that none of the 147 men who engaged in receptive oral intercourse with at least one partner and swallowed semen became infected.

Heterosexual transmission by ordinary penetrative vaginal intercourse is quite possible, and this is the commonest route of transmission in Africa. Where a woman is in a relationship with an infected or high-risk man — a bisexual, an intravenous drug abuser, a transfusion recipient or a haemophiliac — she is at risk. A particular case study was described in the United States where a wife was infected from her bisexual husband with ordinary vaginal intercourse. He subsequently died from *Pneumocystis carinii* pneumonia. She then had a sexual relationship, vaginal intercourse only, with a next-door neighbour, but she subsequently developed AIDS and also died of *Pneumocystis carinii* pneumonia. The neighbour was found to be infected and currently has persistent generalised lymphadenopathy (PGL). So the virus can be passsed from man to woman to man.

It is believed that the virus is more efficiently passed from man to woman than from woman to man, but it is still perfectly possible for a man to be infected by a woman, and infection of men by female prostitutes is thought to play a large role in the heterosexual spread of the infection. In the United States many of those infected in the so-called 'no-risk group' (not homosexuals, drug abusers or transfusion recipients) were found to have multiple prostitute contacts and their infection is attributed to this activity.

The virus is found in semen and in vaginal secretions, and more especially in secretions from the cervix, or neck of the womb. In one of a group of women infected with the virus, no virus was isolated from the vagina or cervix initially, but when the woman was aroused to orgasm the virus was isolated. This suggests that the natural secretion of fluids with sexual arousal may increase the chances of the virus being present, especially if T4 lymphocytes are present in the secretions. Men with a history of previous sexually transmitted diseases have a higher concentration of T4 lymphocytes in their semen.

It is at least theoretically possible for the virus to be transmitted through any body fluid, though it is present in especially high concentrations in semen. The virus has been shown to be present in saliva, but it is highly unlikely that it can be transmitted by kissing. Indeed some experts say that you would need to swallow several pints of saliva before you would be at risk of being infected. Not only is the virus present in very small quantities in saliva, but saliva also has inactivating enzymes that break down the virus. People are sometimes worried that they may be infected through cuts, abrasions and ulcers, both internal and external, but no cases have been documented of transmission of the infection through oral sex, not even where semen was swallowed. All the same, it is not wise to engage in any practices that involve exchange of body fluids (where one person's body fluids are received into the other person's body) and this 'no exchange of body fluids' rule is the safe sex guideline.

The important role of sexual transmission is further confirmed by looking at the age/sex breakdown of those who are predominantly infected. They are from the third and fourth decades, which are the most sexually active age groups (as well as the first and second years of life reflecting infection in the newborn from an infected mother). This same pattern is found in Africa. Some people have wondered whether the disease might not be carried and passed on by insects, such as mosquitoes, but if it were, then we would expect to find infection in all age groups, not just concentrated in a particular age group — it would be curious if the mosquito knew only to bite people who are sexually active. In any case, unlike the malaria virus for instance, which goes through some of its life cycle inside the mosquito, the HIV only grows in human tissue. And even if a mosquito did carry the virus, there would not be enough in its mouthpiece to establish an infection.

The idea of sexual transmission seems to embarrass many people. Many, particularly in the popular press, like to highlight bizarre and unlikely routes of transmission. We should not only face the facts, but make ourselves at ease with the facts. We are lucky that this infection is virtually exclusively transmitted by blood and sex, for therein lies its greatest weakness and our best weapon for containing the spread of infection. It is surely not asking too much of people to be somewhat choosy, and even reticent, when it comes to finding a person with whom to juxtapose their genitals.

THE INFECTION

The virus enters the body and may lie dormant there for many years as a 'provirus' or it may replicate or make more of itself, either slowly or rapidly, with the infected person remaining completely unaware of any changes in themselves and with no signs or symptoms to tell them that they have acquired this infection. The presence of the virus can first be detected at from two weeks to sixteen weeks from the date of acquiring the infection. Antibody, as demonstrated in the HIV antibody test, develops at between four to eight weeks, and is reliably present after twelve weeks.

In 20 per cent of individuals infected a sero-conversion illness is experienced. This is where the patient suffers an illness, rather like many other acute viral illnesses with fever, weakness, headache, joint pains and a measles-like rash with swollen tender glands for a short period of time. It feels similar to a glandular fever syndrome, or the secondary stages of syphilis; yet there is little to distinguish it clearly from a bad influenza or tonsillitis. A small number of people will experience central nervous system involvement with meningitis or encephalitis (inflammation of the brain). These illnesses have a short course of two to three weeks and are associated with the development of the antibodies. However, the majority of infected people give no history of such an illness and either did not have one or had such a mild episode that it was passed off as a common cold.

The infected person then enters a period of latency, where the virus is carried as a provirus by the T4 lymphocyte and either replicates itself very slowly or not at all. The HIV antibody test is positive and some early signs of immune deficiency may be detectable. By and large the patient feels entirely well, and is quite unaware of the infection. Not only are they quite well but they are also fully fit for work, social life, sport and play: and play includes sex play with no diminution of libido (which happens later in the infection) and the full ability to transmit the virus by sex and blood. We do not know how long a person can remain in this condition, or how many will eventually become ill, but we must assume that it can persist for life with continuing potential for infection, and that a percentage of people will go on to get AIDS.

Although most people with HIV infection to date have remained quite well, there is accumulating evidence that with the passage of time people will begin to show signs and symptoms of the infection.

SIGNS AND SYMPTOMS OF HIV INFECTION

Although most people with HIV infection to date have remained quite well, there is accumulating evidence that with the passage of time and if progression of immune deficiency occurs, people will begin to show signs and symptoms of the infection. They may remain well and active, but tell-tale markers begin to appear. We are becoming aware of a broad range of non-lethal conditions that may be recognised as markers for HIV infection. By and large they are not specific to HIV infection, but the manner of their presentation and their persistence and nature may arouse a suspicion of poor immunity, the hallmark of HIV infection.

Persistent generalised lymphadenopathy (PGL)

This was first noted in 1982 in New York amongst homosexual men, and later in other risk groups. It is defined as the occurrence of easily felt enlarged lymph glands of more than

1 centimetre (⅜ ") diameter in at least two or more distinct sites lasting for three months or more. These glands are easily felt in the neck, under the arms and in the groin. They are not painful or tender, they move easily and feel swollen and firm. They may fluctuate in size over short periods of time.

Patients with this condition feel quite well and are usually unaware of its presence. It was discovered to be caused by the HIV when it was found that virtually all patients with this condition were antibody positive. It may last for a short time and the patient then reverts to being an asymptomatic carrier or it may persist for years, or it may progress.

Lymph glands enlarge for many reasons; glands in the neck may enlarge with a sore throat, for instance, and there is generalised glandular swelling with glandular fever, or local glandular swelling with a septic spot. But in persistent generalised lymphadenopathy related to HIV infection, it is a generalised, persistent, glandular swelling of more than three months' duration. If you have had a glandular swelling but are not in a high-risk group you probably have no need to worry, though it would be a good idea to see your doctor anyway to find out what the cause of the swelling is.

AIDS related complex (ARC)

With this condition the patient is *ill* with an HIV infection. It presents as a combination of symptoms, signs and laboratory abnormalities. It is defined as the presence of two or more signs and symptoms and any two or more abnormal laboratory/investigative findings.

Symptoms, signs and laboratory studies in ARC

Symptoms
— Severe malaise (general feeling of being unwell), fatigue, lethargy
— Weight loss (more than 10 per cent of body weight)
— Fever, intermittent or continuous, night sweats
— Unexplained diarrhoea of long duration

Signs
— Persistent generalised lymphadenopathy
— Oral candidiasis (thrush)
— Oral leukoplakia (white plaques on the tongue and lining of the mouth)
— Eczema/folliculitis
— Spleen increases in size

Laboratory studies
— Lymphocytes (>1.5 x 10^9)
— Platelets (>150 x 10^9)
— Anaemia
— T helper cells (>0.40 x 10^9/L) (ratio of T helper/T suppressor inverted)
— Increased serum globulin levels
— Decreased response of lymphocytes to antigens
— Loss of delayed sensitivity reactions on skin testing

ARC could be thought of as a more chronic or later presentation of HIV infection with symptoms. Its signs and symptoms may overlap with those of the opportunistic infections seen in full AIDS. Clinically the patient is usually quite unwell with profound tiredness and malaise. Waking hours may be constantly interrupted by diarrhoea; sleeping by night sweats. The patient is usually apprehensive and anxious, often depressed, always fearful that they have or will shortly have AIDS. This is a reasonable fear as patients with ARC show a much greater rate of progression to AIDS, and indeed some people call this condition pre-AIDS.

Because the signs and symptoms in ARC and AIDS are non-specific these conditions are easily confused with other illnesses, so doctors looking after the case have to seek assiduously for the presence of opportunistic infections and tumours, which would confirm the diagnosis.

Skin manifestations of infection
There is a wide range of changes on the skin in HIV-infected patients, often quite common conditions that are expressed in a more florid and persistent manner in HIV-infected people.

Seborrhoeic dermatitis is a very common condition in the

population as a whole with dryness, scaling and redness of the skin, particularly on areas of the body that skin scales from the scalp may fall upon, eyebrows, cheeks, shoulders, upper arms and chest, as well as in body folds. It is sometimes mistaken for dandruff which is an intensification of the normal process of losing skin scales, but in seborrhoeic dermatitis the loss of skin scales is abnormally increased. It presents as a minor slightly irritating condition and sometimes quite florid. In the HIV-infected person, however, it becomes much more florid and serves as a clue for diagnosis. If it is very severe and extensive it may indicate a greater degree of immuno-suppression with a greater chance of progression to AIDS.

Folliculitis is an inflammatory condition of the numerous glandular areas or follicles, including hair follicles, which occur in the skin. It develops as small inflamed spots which often are intensely itching or burning. They occur at the sites mentioned above but also extend beyond these areas onto the abdomen, thighs and under the arm pits. It is often seen in the beard area and is made worse by shaving. The yeast *Pithrosporum orbicularae* has been identified in skin scrapings. The condition is often resistant to treatment in HIV-infected patients and the itchiness can cause considerable distress. Skin infections are common, especially by the herpes viruses. Shingles, caused by the *Herpes zoster* virus, occurs in about 25 per cent of ARC and AIDS patients. Initial infection with this virus causes chickenpox, and shingles represents a reactivation of a latent infection in a host. Again the condition would tend to be more extensive, florid and prolonged; and recurrences are not uncommon, which is most unusual in the normal person. Its occurrence probably relates to the progression of the immuno-suppression and is a poor prognostic sign. *Herpes simplex* virus causing 'cold sores' on the lips and genitalia reactivate more frequently and have a more florid and prolonged course. In particular peri-anal herpes can cause substantial distress and discomfort, particularly if the patient has diarrhoea. This persists for weeks or months as opposed to the usual ten-to-twenty-day course of this infection. It can be treated with Acyclovir which gives considerable relief and maintenance therapy is often required. If the herpes infection disseminates to other parts of the body and the patient is HIVab+, then it constitutes an opportunistic infection and the case becomes one of AIDS.

Warts caused by the human papilloma virus often present, either by reactivation of a pre-existing infection or by a new infection. They grow profusely, particularly in the warm, moist genital areas and may occur in unusual sites such as the mouth.

Other superficial skin infections, such as cellulitis, athlete's foot, impetigo, paronychia and *Molluscum contagiosum* occur more commonly in a more florid and persistent way. Greying of the hair and diffuse hair loss together with weight loss give an appearance of rapid aging. The skin in infected patients may also become very dry and scaly. Pre-existing skin conditions such as psoriasis may become more florid.

Oral manifestations of infection
Coating of the tongue is so common as to be of little diagnostic help but is frequently seen in HIV-infected patients. Oral thrush or *Candida* infection is very common with large plaques of white material on the lining of the mouth which can be scraped off. Occasionally the lining is just red. It is a poor prognostic sign. The angles of the mouth sometimes become sore with angular stomatitis.

Hairy leukoplakia is a condition unique to HIV-infected patients and is seen as white lesions on the sides and underside of the tongue. The microscopic appearances show changes typical of wart virus infection (HPV) and whorls of keratin giving a hairy appearance, and electron microscopy shows particles of the Epstein Barr virus. They may regress spontaneously but again this is associated with a poor prognosis.

Mouth ulcers and inflammation are non-specific findings which are common in these patients, and may be very severe. Teeth may be more prone to problems especially dental abscesses and gum recession. The mouth is often the first place where intestinal Kaposi's sarcoma becomes apparent.

Other manifestations of infection
Sinusitis, nasal discharge and catarrh are very common in HIV-infected patients. The problem may be more prolonged and

often causes a severe persisting headache. Cancer of the anus and rectum has been noted to occur more commonly in gay men and may be associated with genital wart virus infection. Its presentation in HIV-infected patients is more frequent. Reactivation of tuberculosis that had been lying dormant has been reported, and syphilis may also be reactivated.

Non-specific behavioural changes are reported in up to 60 per cent of the people infected in America, but to a lesser extent in England and Europe. Initially it was only detected with sophisticated psychological testing, but as it progresses it may become quite marked with blunting of concentration and memory, apathy and depression. Libido is also lost. It can be difficult to discern whether these changes are secondary to primary infection of the brain or are caused by the psychological strain of the infection.

In Africa a common manifestation of this infection is 'slim disease' where there is gross loss of weight secondary to diarrhoea from gastrointestinal tract infection, with aging and apathy.

PROGRESSION TO AIDS

The great enigma of this infection is how many people will progress to AIDS and over what period of time. We need to know what, if any, are the factors that pre-dispose towards progression. Does progression occur at a constant rate over a period of time, and is there any end point in time to it? We do not yet know much about progression to other equally lethal conditions, such as HIV encephalopathy and the potential for cancer to develop in infected individuals either. The long latent period between the time of acquiring the infection and presentation with AIDS makes an accurate projection difficult at this stage of our knowledge of the disease.

Numerous studies have been carried out and have reported a range of progression from 6.4 per cent in five years to 34 per cent in three years. One has even predicted that 75 per cent will progress to AIDS.

The important thing to remember when dealing with these figures is that they may not be related to the length of time the infection was present, as they are often taken from small highly selected populations and may not be representative of infected groups as a whole. Bias may be introduced by 'volunteers' taking part in studies because they feel themselves to be particularly at risk, in the hope that they will get additional medical support by being involved.

In a multicentre study report in *Science* in 1985, 34 per cent of infected homosexual men progressed to AIDS in Manhattan over three years. Seventeen per cent did so in Washington and 8 per cent in Denmark. The intravenous drug abusing group had a 25 per cent incidence and the haemophiliac group 13 per cent over three years. The significantly higher incidence in Manhattan gay men was thought to be related to a longer duration of the infection at the time of enrolment into the study. In those people where the timing of the infection was known by the appearance of HIVab+, it was suggested that AIDS in adults usually develops more than two years after infection and that new cases continue to appear more than five years later.

Another three-year prospective study of HIV infection in gay men, carried out in London, showed that 13 per cent have progressed to AIDS, 42 per cent to PGL and only 48 per cent remained fully well and symptom free. Progression to AIDS was significantly associated with concurrent infection with other sexually transmitted diseases.

The MACS (Multicentre AIDS Cohort Study) yielded a group of 1835 homosexual men who were HIVab+ at the time of entry to the study. The subsequent development of AIDS in fifty-nine men was reported recently. The chance of progression to AIDS each year was expressed as a percentage: 2.6 per cent of asymptomatic men, 3.2 per cent in men with PGL and 8.6 per cent in those with ARC at their first visits, progressed to AIDS per annum. They found that history of sex with someone with AIDS, or in whom AIDS subsequently developed, was significantly associated with the development of AIDS. This is somewhat intriguing as it may suggest the possibility that some strains of HIV are more virulent than others. On the other hand it may simply be a marker of longer duration of infection, since those cases whose partners have had HIV infection long enough to develop AIDS were exposed to it for a longer period of time. A reducing level of HIVab was also noted to be a significant predictor of progression.

However, a major limitation of the MACS study is that the duration of infection in HIVab+ people who entered the study was unknown, and that it will require further prospective studies to determine more clearly the effective duration of infection. No relationship was seen with the number of partners, their age, race, frequency of anal intercourse or use of nitrites (poppers) in the preceding two years.

In another recent study in New York, a small group of homosexual men with thrombocytopenia or loss of platelets required for blood clotting, were observed for approximately three years. They were noted to have the same expected incidence of AIDS as other gay men in Manhattan (36 per cent). The authors gave evidence to support the theory that the risk of developing AIDS was not constant, but increased with time. If it was assumed that the risk was constant, the number of cases in the first two to three years will be over-estimated and under-estimated thereafter. The pattern was interpreted as that of increasing risk with the passage of time.

It should be borne in mind that these studies were carried out in samples of gay men who are predominantly white and well educated. There are no comparable studies amongst the black populations in America or Africa, or amongst intravenous drug abusers, although evidence to date suggests that the figures would be comparable.

Pregnancy increases greatly the chances of progression to AIDS and high rates of progression are also seen among the newborn. Our existing knowledge indicates that the length of time a person is infected is the major determinant in the progression to AIDS and that there is no evidence of any decline in the rate of progression after a period of years. In fact, one model shows an increasing rate with the passage of time.

ACQUIRED IMMUNE DEFICIENCY SYNDROME (AIDS)

AIDS itself is a life-threatening syndrome of conditions opportunistic in patients whose immunity has been impaired by the HIV infection. This is the most severe form of the infection and was the first form to be recognised and defined.

The prognosis for AIDS is bad, with 80 per cent of patients being dead within two years. The outlook for those with opportunistic infections like *Pneumocystis carinii* pneumonia is much worse, with only a 4 per cent two-year survival rate compared to Kaposi's sarcoma which has a 22 per cent two-year survival rate. For those who do survive for three years or more, the outlook becomes quite good, but that may be because the original diagnosis was incorrect. Patients often experience a series of opportunistic infections over a six-to-eighteen-month period before a final fatal episode.

Pneumocystis carinii pneumonia is the commonest presentation in the western world. It may occur at any stage and in patients with other opportunistic infections. A further 20-25 per cent present with Kaposi's sarcoma and these are predominantly homosexual cases. The remainder of cases have a presentation in the central nervous system, gastrointestinal tract or a tumour.

Chest presentations

The lungs are the most frequently involved organ in AIDS, most commonly with *Pneumocystis carinii* pneumonia. The condition presents with a dry cough with a progressive loss of breath. It generally comes on over two to six weeks but may take a much longer time and occasionally only a very short time. Chest pains, like pleurisy, are seen in some cases and this is particularly sore on coughing or on taking in a deep breath. Fever is always present, usually low grade but accompanied with night sweats. Often there is little to be found on examination except an increase in the rate of respiration and sometimes crackling sounds at the base of the lungs.

Chest X-rays may show some changes, but it is important to appreciate that X-rays may show nothing in the early stages of the infection where the immuno-depression damps down the normal inflammatory response. Definitive diagnosis may be made by obtaining a specimen of lung tissue by bronchoscopy, which involves putting a flexible tube down into the lung. This is then examined by microscopy after special staining for the cysts of *Pneumocystis carinii*.

Pneumocystis carinii pneumonia may be treated with

antibiotics and survival per episode of the disease has improved with prompt diagnosis and treatment. This stresses the importance of early diagnosis by early bronchoscopy, with the recognition of the importance of quite subtle signs and symptoms in at-risk patients. The infection can 'flare out of control' in a few days if not treated. Most survive after the initial satisfactorily treated first episode, but recurrences within a matter of months are common. Many will survive for six to twelve months, but only 4 per cent survive for two years.

Other infections such as cytomegalovirus may cause primary infection in the lung causing an atypical pneumonia that clinically frequently resembles *Pneumocystis carinii* pneumonia. Unusual cubical bacilli infections, such as *Mycobacterium avium intra-cellulare* (MAI), have been reported in the United States and in England an increasing number of cases of ordinary tuberculosis (TB) have been seen. It is hard to know if this reflects a reactivation of latent infection present or fresh infection with an organism that is common in the environment.

Kaposi's sarcoma may occur in the lungs and is more likely to be localised. Only a small proportion of the patients have symptoms, but autopsy findings indicate that many patients have pulmonary (lung) Kaposi's sarcoma.

Gastrointestinal presentations

AIDS affects the gastrointestinal tract, which is the tract from the mouth to the anus along which food is ingested, absorbed and excreted. The symptoms are of weight loss and diarrhoea, whatever the site or type of infection, and one has to search diligently for a wide variety of different organisms to make a definitive diagnosis. The problem is often how to distinguish between the diarrhoea/wasting seen in ARC from that seen in AIDS, and exhaustive investigations are required, often repeatedly, to make the diagnosis of the opportunistic infection.

The very common yeast *Candida albicans* normally colonises the gastrointestinal tract and may cause annoying superficial infection such as vaginal thrush. Those who suffer recurrent 'thrush' are often thought to have a minor impairment of their immune system and *Candida* infection is common throughout the course of HIV infection as mentioned previously in the section on ARC.

To enter the category of an 'opportunistic infection' characteristic of AIDS, *Candida* must be present in a disseminated form and not just present as localised plaques in the mouth or vaginal thrush. It may spread down the gastrointestinal tract to the oesophagus and sometimes the stomach. It may be symptomless, but often causes an aching discomfort on swallowing food or drink. It is diagnosed by an X-ray examination. The possibility that candidiasis of the small bowel may cause the malabsorption and diarrhoea symptoms seen in AIDS has been raised. The infection can be held at bay with appropriate long-term local applications or a systemic drug for disseminated infection.

A small parasite, Cryptosporidium, has been a known cause of diarrhoea in cattle, but it has only recently been reported as affecting humans, usually causing a short, self-limiting episode of diarrhoea.

It causes a profuse watery diarrhoea which persists in AIDS. The parasite is identified by special staining and microscopy of the bowel motion. There is no effective treatment and patients only survive a matter of months, despite intensive supportive therapy. The high-volume diarrhoea causes considerable nursing and social problems.

Localised herpes infection in the peri-anal area was mentioned in the section on HIV infection. It persists and becomes more florid in AIDS patients and if it becomes extensive or disseminated, persisting for more than one month, it will constitute an opportunistic infection for the diagnosis of AIDS. A florid, persistent peri-anal ulcer (or ulcers) is seen, often with swelling resembling external 'piles' for which they are often mistaken by the patient. Defecation (opening the bowels) is particularly painful and if the patient also has diarrhoea causes considerable debility and distress, both physically and psychologically. Fortunately it usually responds to the anti-herpes drug, Acyclovir. Extensive ulcerating lesions may need to be examined by biopsy to exclude cancer of the anus and rectum, which is seen more commonly in immuno-suppressed patients.

The peri-oral herpes infection may be more extensive than normal but rarely produces the florid presentation seen in the peri-anal area.

Cytomegalovirus (CMV) is common in HIV-infected patients and it is identified by its characteristic inclusion body seen on microscopy. In the gastrointestinal tract it may cause an oesophagitis or infection of the swallowing tube, clinically indistinguishable from that described for *Candida*, except for more severe symptoms and some low-grade fever.

In the large bowel it may cause a CMV colitis with recurrent watery diarrhoea accompanied by blood. There is fever, and tenderness and distension of the stomach and X-rays show distended loops of bowels. Diagnosis is by biopsy and the virus may be isolated. In a more chronic form, chronic diarrhoea and weight loss will occur.

Kaposi's sarcoma primarily appears as skin lesions, but in AIDS patients the gastrointestinal tract is commonly involved and lesions may be seen on the palate in most cases. Usually the condition is silent and Kaposi's sarcoma nodules may be found on any part of the gastrointestinal tract. Some cases, however, have a more aggressive form of Kaposi's sarcoma and the wall of the gut would be infiltrated leading to colicky pain, ulceration and bleeding with the late development of a constriction of the bowel leading to intestinal obstruction.

Patients with immune deficiency are particularly susceptible to infection with the typhoid bacillus, *Salmonella typhimurium*, as this bacterium is normally dealt with by the cellular immune system. This has been seen more commonly in England and is associated with eating battery-raised poultry in which this organism is common. It is recommended that HIV-infected patients should avoid this type of food product and be sure that their food is well cooked. Other enteric infections which have been described commonly in gay men, such as *Giardia lamblia* and *Entamoeba histolytica*, appear to pose no special risks for the patient with HIV infection who deals with these organisms in the normal way.

Central nervous system presentations
The brain was originally noted to be a major site for

opportunistic infections and for unusual growths of B-cells, a B-cell lymphoma. Again, signs of the disease may be atypical depending on the ability of the host's immune response. They may be either related to localised space occupying lesions — focal: or widespread in the central nervous system — diffuse. The back of the eye, the retina, allows a window on what is going on in the brain.

Recognition that the brain may be a site of primary HIV infection resulting in HIV encephalopathy has added another dimension to the picture, and obviously makes it more difficult to know whether early changes are due to primary infection or to opportunistic infection. As opportunistic infections may be treatable, a full investigation is required.

HIV encephalopathy seems to be caused directly by the virus itself, in contrast to most of the other illnesses suffered by AIDS patients, which are opportunistic infections and tumours that get a hold on the body because the immune system is defective. HIV encephalopathy can occur, however, in HIV-infected people even if their immune system is still relatively undamaged, and they have not progressed to ARC or AIDS. It can also present in AIDS. Ten per cent of AIDS patients present with neurological problems and there are neurological findings in 40 per cent of patients with AIDS. At post mortem examinations 70 per cent of AIDS patients show abnormality in the central nervous system.

Encephalopathy is a condition of the brain, and it presents as a dementia complex. It starts off with very subtle changes in concentration, memory and alertness. It may be accompanied by depression, lethargy, withdrawal and loss of libido. These early changes may be quite difficult to see and even under psychological testing difficult to measure. They may be best noticed by friends, relatives or lovers, who see a change in mood and personality and by workmates who note a deterioration in work patterns.

As the condition progresses the changes may become more marked with loss of verbal fluency, dizziness and poor muscle co-ordination. The ability to perform tasks at work and even to drive a car may be impaired. Epileptic fits may also occur. The effects become more stereotyped as the disease progresses and eventually the patient ends up with a total dementia with inability to respond to simple questions except by one-word responses: immobile, bedridden and incontinent.

Examination by computer axial tomography (CAT) scan shows wasting away of the brain, especially the white matter, with widening of the fluid-filled spaces, the ventricles. A similar picture may be caused by some of the opportunistic infections, which may be treatable, so it is important to carry out a full investigation including an examination of the cerebral spinal fluid, the fluid bathing the brain and spinal cord to exclude these conditions.

A corollary has been drawn between HIV producing this encephalopathy and the visna virus that causes encephalopathy in sheep. The visna virus lies dormant in sheep for ten to fifteen years. It then activates and causes a fatal encephalopathy. It is possible that the same thing may happen with the HIV. The fear that a large proportion of HIV-infected people, who number in excess of one million in the United States alone, could go on to this condition has been expressed and our health services and social structure are unlikely to be able to deal with a problem of this magnitude.

A peripheral neuropathy has been described where the nerves to the peripheral parts of the body have been directly affected. It may occur in HIV-infected persons as well as those with full AIDS. Symptoms include alteration in sensation, as well as feelings of tingling, burning and even pain. Muscle weakness may be the presenting feature and is localised to particular groups of muscles at a time.

Some opportunistic infections cause localised lesions or abscesses in the brain. Initially the patient appears just tired, lethargic and confused. Then the signs and symptoms will be dependent upon the site of the lesion, which may be multiple. Headache and dizziness may also present accompanied by limb weakness or paralysis: epileptic attacks may occur. The commonest cause is *Toxoplasma gondi* which is a common organism in domestic pets causing transient glandular swelling in the immuno-competent patient and is dealt with by the cellular immune system. Other causes include *Candida* abscesses and a primary B-cell lymphoma, a growth of lymphoid-derived cells in the brain.

The lesions may be seen on CAT scan and are often seen with a ring effect around them due to surrounding swelling of brain tissue. There is an antibody test for toxoplasmosis but diagnosis cannot be made on the basis of a single test, or excluded by a negative one. Treatment is available and it is often thought worthwhile to treat a mass lesion as a toxoplasma abscess to assess response. Toxoplasmosis is also seen as a retinitis (see below) which does not need to occur concurrently with a brain lesion.

The fungus *Cryptococcus neoformans* commonly infects the cerebral spinal fluid and causes meningitis. Symptoms include headache, fever, weight loss, nausea and vomiting with few signs of meningeal irritation, such as neck stiffness. There may also be a decrease in concentration and memory. Diagnosis is made by taking a spinal tap and examining the spinal fluid by special staining for evidence of the fungus.

Rarely a diffuse encephalitis (inflammation of the brain) may be caused by other organisms, including *Herpes simplex*, cytomegalovirus, atypical mycobacterium, a diffuse lymphocytic infiltration, and by progressive multifocal leuko-encephalopathy, which is an unusual demyelinating disease (a disease that attacks the nerve fibres) caused by a virus and resulting in widespread central nervous system signs.

Clinically the retina (back of the eyeball) is very useful as it allows direct observation into the optic nerve and optic artery, giving a reflection of conditions within the skull.

'Cotton wool spots' occur frequently in patients with AIDS or in HIV-infected persons. They rarely interfere with vision and regress spontaneously over a period of five to six weeks. Cytomegalovirus retinitis causes inflammation of the retina and is the frequent cause of loss of vision. This is an ophthalmic emergency and immediate assessment should be made. It may progress to blindness if it occurs in both eyes.

Skin presentations
Kaposi's sarcoma is the second commonest presentation of AIDS and is best thought of as an opportunistic tumour. It occurs almost exclusively in the homosexual risk group and some people think that there may be another virus or infectious

agent which causes Kaposi's sarcoma and is expressed in the immuno-suppressed patient. The degree of immuno-suppression seen in patients with Kaposi's sarcoma alone is often not as profound as seen with other opportunistic infections. Patients with Kaposi's sarcoma alone have a better prognosis, but those with Kaposi's sarcoma accompanied by an opportunistic infection have a very poor prognosis.

Classic Kaposi's sarcoma is a tumour usually occurring in elderly people of Mediterranean and African stock, affecting the skin, especially on the legs and feet. It pursues a rather benign course growing slowly and is non-invasive. It is rarely life-threatening.

The epidemic form of Kaposi's sarcoma in AIDS patients is quite different. Here it occurs in young people in a very aggressive form and nearly 80 per cent are dead in two years. The new occurrence of this form of the disease in clusters of homosexual men was one of the first signals that alerted us to AIDS. This epidemic form is not localised to one area of the body, such as the legs, as is common in classical Kaposi's sarcoma. Skin presentation has the advantage of being easily observed and allows medical attention to be sought early in the course of the condition.

The lesions of Kaposi's sarcoma are actual tumours and are felt sometimes before they are seen. They are seen as firm slightly raised lumps, not tender, which grow in size over the course of a few weeks, but they seldom exceed two inches in diameter. The lesions may present in the classical distribution on the lower legs, but more commonly they occur scattered widely all over the body, and often silently inside the body. Often individual lesions may go away by themselves, but they rarely all regress spontaneously. The skin lesions of Kaposi's sarcoma may resemble a wide variety of common benign skin conditions, so in at-risk patients anxiety is common and it is usually necessary to make a definitive diagnosis by taking a tiny fragment of the suspicious spot or area (biopsy) and subjecting it to examination by microscope. A distinct pattern of spinical cells and red blood cells outside the blood vessels can be seen. The prognosis depends upon the degree of immuno-deficiency and can be quite good where a moderate number of T4 lymphocytes remain. Treatment is evolving but one must be careful not to use any therapy that in an attempt to kill or poison the KS cells, such as cytotoxic therapy, could also poison the immune system and hasten the progression of the immuno-deficiency. For this reason one often just observes cases of Kaposi's sarcoma and hopes for regression, or deals with isolated lesions by surgical removal or local radio-therapy. However, when the disease is more widespread, treatment has less to offer and the outlook is worse.

The range of skin conditions and infections as described in the section on HIV infection can also occur in patients with AIDS, although shingles is less common. Skin lesions may occur with widespread infections, particularly with fungi and protozoa, and the lesions are often unusual, requiring biopsy for diagnosis.

Glandular presentations
Some cases of AIDS may present with swollen lymph glands only. This may be due to spreading infection, such as opportunistic fungi or bacilli or infiltration with growths such as Kaposi's sarcoma or lymphomas. This is different from the persistent generalised lymphadenopathy (PGL) seen in earlier stages of HIV infection: the glands are not symmetrically enlarged and often they may be matted together. Diagnosis may be made by biopsy of one of the nodes.

Non-Hodgkins lymphoma or growth of the lymphoid tissue has been newly seen in homosexual men. They have very aggressive B-cell growth occurring in a number of sites where one does not normally see lymphoid tissue. Epstein Barr virus has been implicated as a cause of a similar lymphoma in Africa, Burkitt's lymphoma, where it was observed to be transmitted by insect vectors. Homosexual men frequently show evidence of exposure to Epstein Barr virus and it is thought by some that a depressed immune surveillance may allow the cancer producing potential of this virus to be expressed. It is also associated with nasopharyngeal (nose and throat) cancer, which is being seen more commonly in HIV-infected people.

HIV INFECTION, AIDS AND PREGNANCY

Although the 'AIDS epidemic' as we see it in the western world is mainly a male phenomenon, the infection is readily acquired by women. Heterosexual transmission is the major route in Africa and it is becoming increasingly important in the western world, through intravenous drug abuse or through sex with bisexual men, who constitute about 10 per cent of the homosexual population and are often secretive about their activities, especially if married. Other women at risk would include prostitutes, sexual contacts of infected men, and those whose sexual partners are in a high-risk group and those with multiple sexual partners.

The consequences for a woman infected with the HIV of getting pregnant are immense. Not only does she stand a 60-70 per cent chance of having an infected baby, but also her chances of progressing to AIDS herself are substantially increased to approximately 50 per cent.

In pregnancy the immune system is naturally suppressed to ensure that the mother does not reject the foetus. While the immune system is suppressed a mother may be susceptible to genital warts or to thrush, and this physiological immuno-suppression in pregnancy may act as a co-factor in bringing on AIDS in a woman who is already HIV-infected.

At present any woman who is found to be infected should be strongly advised regarding the dangers of becoming pregnant both to herself and the baby. As we learn more about this disease we may be able to help women in this position, but for the moment the infected girl must be strongly counselled against pregnancy, helped to adjust her lifestyle and expectations to this fact and given contraceptive support. There does not seem to be much point in general ante-natal screening, as by the time the woman is pregnant it is too late, and pre-marital screening may not be a great deal of use either, as many unmarried women become pregnant.

Current evidence shows that transmission to the newborn takes place before birth and the virus has been isolated from foetuses at twenty-four and thirty weeks' gestation. Intervention by Caesarean section has not affected the rate of infection. Breast milk has also been implicated in the transmission of the infection and HIV-infected mothers should not breast-feed their babies or donate milk to milk banks.

There is evidence of congenital abnormalities being increased following infection with HIV at present, the infection itself may cause abnormalities like microcephaly (small head) and facial abnormalities.

Men who are infected or in a high-risk group with female partners should be advised of these facts and their partners should be offered involvement in counselling. Men who donate sperm should be screened for HIV infection as it has been shown to be transmitted by artificial insemination by donor (AID). It is now current practice to store donated sperm for three months and not to use it until the donor has been tested negative three months after the donation.

Since so many of the public will be unaware of these risks and factors pertaining to them, it is essential that they are informed through public health education so that they can identify themselves, preferably before they get pregnant. We cannot expect people to act responsibly if we do not take the responsibility for informing them.

HIV INFECTION AND AIDS IN CHILDREN

HIV-infected children are either born to infected mothers or acquire the infection through blood transfusion. Studies throughout the world, including Dublin, show a 60-70 per cent rate of transmission from an infected mother to her baby in the womb.

Paediatric HIV infection carries a higher risk of progression to AIDS in a shorter time than in the adult. Preliminary studies indicate that up to 50 per cent of infected babies may develop AIDS within two years. In the first year of life the immune system is bombarded with new foreign antigens which it learns to recognise and builds up an antibody response. The T-cells are at a higher state of activation which may act as a co-factor for the virus to reproduce itself.

In the first few months of life a baby is protected by its mother's antibodies and the maternal antibody supplies are replenished through breast-feeding. This carry-over of maternal antibodies makes diagnosis in the newborn difficult, as practically all babies born of infected mothers will be positive from the carry-over. Consequently a positive HIVab test at birth does not tell you that the baby is infected — it tells you that the baby may be infected but the mother certainly was infected. One has to repeat the HIVab test at six months, by which time the maternal antibodies will have disappeared, and if it is persistently present this means that the baby is infected. If it is found to be negative, it means that the baby has escaped infection in most cases. (Other ways of making the diagnosis of infection in the first months of life would include a positive viral culture from the infant at risk or use of a newly developed antigen test which directly detects viral proteins in the sample. A further technique is being developed of *in situ* 'hybridisation' of labelled HIV specific DNA to cultured lymphocytes from an infant.)

Low birth weight, failure to thrive, fever, frequent bacterial infections and increased susceptibility to diarrhoea are common symptoms in babies. Often the head is of smaller size, microcephalic. Many children present later with a chronic lymphoid pneumonitis with recurrent chest infections. It is diagnosed by lung biopsy. There is some indication that these children may have a better prognosis. Frank AIDS usually involves the opportunistic infections and Kaposi's sarcoma is very rarely seen in children. There may also be progressive and unexplained neurological deterioration, including late onset of seizures, lack of development, cessation of brain growth and a diffuse encephalopathy.

These children will pose considerable social and caring problems. If they are very ill, as a proportion of them are, they may require institutional care and there may be soiling from high-volume diarrhoea, vomiting as well as urine to be dealt with.

These would only pose a danger to health-care workers or family members where gross breaches of hygiene occurred: only one such incident has been reported, where a child infected from a blood transfusion infected his mother. Institutional care may also be required where the parents are incapable of caring for the child through illness or because of their lifestyle in the case of intravenous drug abusers. Often their parents die of

AIDS and the children become 'AIDS orphans'. Potential foster parents are found to be very reluctant to adopt these children who are then often left in institutional care as AIDS orphans. Some children are caught in an 'antibody trap' where because of maternal antibody transfer they are HIVab positive themselves at birth and it is not until the test is repeated after six months that one can see that they are free of infection. Obviously a reliable test for early diagnosis would be a substantial help to these children.

Section II

CHAPTER 3
THE PROBLEM IN IRELAND

In some respects Ireland was ill-prepared and ill-equipped to deal with the AIDS epidemic. Our facilities for the control of sexually transmitted diseases were lamentable in the 1970s and early 1980s. They consisted of part-time clinics run by part-time personnel, poorly staffed and equipped, with no contact-tracing facilities, save that done on the patient's own initiative. Facilities for the treatment of the intravenous drug abusers were even less adequate with a small detoxification unit in Jervis Street Hospital serving the entire country and an out-patient referral unit in the hospital. In the early 1980s it was estimated that there were something in the region of 3000-5000 people abusing intravenous drugs in Dublin alone. They frequently turned to stealing, prostitution and pushing drugs to feed their expensive habit. It was not until parents became aware of what was happening to their children that neighbourhood campaigns to drive out the pushers began and that the tide started to turn and numbers involved in drug abuse began to fall.

Ireland is a small country with a tight-knit social structure with strong rural ties. Despite superficial appearances, social and sexual reticence is the order of the day for most people, though the bright lights of Leeson Street and the escapes of Greece and Spain may induce some temporary relaxation of these strictures for some, and one can never neglect the strong influence of alcohol on the inhibitions.

In caring for individual cases so far, families and friends have shown great individual care, understanding and love for the patient, which often meant that he could be cared for at home surrounded by his relatives and friends. Fortunately, we have never had a situation in this country where a person with AIDS was put out 'on the streets', which has happened in societies less compassionate than our own. In my experience common sense has always prevailed and when one explains that the infection is transmitted solely by blood and sex, people readily lose their fears about any danger to themselves from day-to-day living and caring for people.

AIDS CASES
The first cases of AIDS presented in Ireland in 1982. They were both homosexuals with Kaposi's sarcoma. One is known to have died; the other left the country and is presumed to have died. They both contracted their infections outside Ireland.

AIDS CASES — IRELAND

1982	1983	1984	1985	1986	To 30/4 1987
IVDA					
				Paediatric ●	
				Paediatric ●	●
				PCP ● +	●
HAEMOPHILIAC					●
		PCP ●	PCP ● +	● +	●
HOMOSEXUAL					
KS □ +		PCP □ +	KS ●		
KS □ +	KS □ +	KS □ +	TP ● +	B cell L ● +	●

□ probably acquired abroad
● probably acquired in Ireland
+ died

PCP = Pneumocystis carinii pneumonia
KS = Kaposi's sarcoma
TP = toxoplasmosis
B cell L = B cell lymphoma.

A further case returned to Ireland from abroad in 1983. Three further cases were reported in 1984: one was a haemophiliac and is alive, the other two contracted their infections abroad. Three cases were reported in 1985: one was a haemophiliac and the other two were homosexual and would have had the opportunity to acquire the infection either in Ireland or abroad and so represented the first appearance of potential indigenous infection in Ireland. One of these patients is still alive and under treatment.

The figures in 1986 almost doubled, with a further five cases being notified. One was a homosexual and could have contracted his infection either here or abroad and has subsequently died, and one was a haemophiliac. For the first time in that year there was official reporting of cases relating to intravenous drug abuse. Three cases presented, one case of *Pneumocystis carinii* pneumonia, and there were two paediatric cases of AIDS, children of mothers who were intravenous drug abusers. A further five cases have been notified so far for 1987 at time of going to press (May 1987), more than one a month. One is homosexual, two are intravenous drug abusers and two are haemophiliacs.

The trickle of cases from 1983 is turning to a steady stream. The initial cases were from the homosexual risk group, which was probably the first group to be infected. Cases from this risk group remain sporadic and are too few in number to show any discernible trends. The first haemophiliac case was seen in 1984, but it was not until 1985/6 that a definite pattern of haemophilia progression to AIDS was noted. This appears to be building up with some consistency. Intravenous drug abusing related cases did not appear as a sole factor risk group until 1986. It is likely that the infection entered this group in 1983/4 and we are now beginning to see cases of AIDS emerge.

To date all the cases have been in males and the overall mortality rate has been 55 per cent. Reporting of cases is done on a voluntary basis to the Department of Health and they are dealt with in a confidential manner. It is not necessary to give details which would identify the patient; it is solely required to report the case. Overall it would appear that reporting has been good over the past two years and that most of the medical profession are aware of the condition now and of its public health importance.

HIV-INFECTED CASES — ANTIBODY POSITIVE

Actual AIDS cases represent only the 'tip of the iceberg'. It is the end stage of the infection with a high mortality, representing only a small percentage of those infected at any given time, and developing only with the passage of considerable time. It does not give any real indication of the current state of infection in a community. However, the number of people infected can be gauged by the results of the HIV antibody test. This is carried out by the Virus Reference Laboratory. It is offered to all who need it and is available through the STD clinics, the drug unit at Jervis Street Hospital and GPs. It is carried out in hospitals, where appropriate, as part of a patient's care and investigation. This test is usually and should always be carried out with a person's informed consent.

Blood donations are all routinely tested for HIVab+, and donors are informed of this before they make their donation. It is assumed that making the donation implies consent to the test. However, giving blood should not be seen as a way of getting yourself tested: it is extremely important that those who are at risk or feel themselves at risk to this infection do not donate blood, as there is a very small chance of an infected donation not being picked up if it is within the first three months 'incubating' stage. Most people in high-risk groups appreciate this and have ceased donating blood. One can only express the highest degree of contempt for one who uses the blood donating clinics as under-cover HIV-testing stations. Not only is a person who does this taking a chance of putting others at risk if they are infected at a stage where the antibody test would not pick up the infection, but they are also depriving themselves of the confidential service provided by other agencies and the pre- and post-test counselling.

Up to the end of March 1987, 8705 people had been tested for HIV antibody in Ireland, and 581 have been found to be positive — 6.6 per cent. The overwhelming majority of these have been associated with particular risk groups and the breakdown is shown below:

HIVab POSITIVITY IN IRELAND TO 31/3/87

Group	Number Tested	Number Positive	% Positive
Intravenous Drug Abusers	1880	364 (276 M) (84 F)	19
Babies of IV Drug Abusers	34	23	68
Homosexuals/Bisexuals	1080	58	5.4
Haemophiliacs	510	107	21
Non-Categorised	5201	25	0.004
Total	8705	581	6.6

Source: Virus Reference Laboratory, UCD

INTRAVENOUS DRUG ABUSERS
Number tested: 1880 — HIVab+ 364 (276m, 84f) — 19%

This group has the highest number of people infected. Infection comes from sharing needles, and there is also the potential for sexual transmission within the group. We have no basic demographic information about the number of people who have taken drugs by injection in Ireland over the past five years, so we don't know how representative the above figures are. They are mainly derived from attenders at the drug unit and from those in prison.

Data on retrospective random testing on blood samples stored from this population from hepatitis B screening would indicate that the infection entered this group in 1982/3 and was firmly established by 1984.

RETROSPECTIVE AND RANDOM HIVab TEST
on intravenous drug abusers

Year	No. Tested	No. Positive	Percentage
1982	88	—	—
1983	59	4	7
1984	34	8	24
1985	473	122	26
1986	749	179	24

Knowledge of this was not available until 1985/6 so little could be done until then to inform people of the even greater and almost inevitable lethal consequences of the habit. However, drug abusers are very resistant to changing their behaviour. They require support, counselling and cajoling by people they can relate to within their own community. They respond to those who seek to help them. Intravenous drug abusers are sexually active, often in stable caring monogamous relationships, but those who do not have stable relationships may seek sexual fulfilment from multiple sexual partners, in some cases amounting to several a week or hundreds over the course of a few years. Prostitution is an easy way for drug abusers to make money quickly to feed their habit. They are addicted to the quick high of drugs, and so they are willing to risk a rapid depreciation of their capital, themselves, to achieve this.

This is an obvious risk to the community at large. The prostitution turned to may be homosexual or heterosexual. Studies throughout the western world have associated HIV infection substantially more with occasional prostitutes who abuse drugs than those who are professional 'pros'. The professional will make her partner use condoms, to protect herself and to protect the client, as after all infections are bad for business and prostitutes are in business. The gifted amateur or the intravenous drug abuser seeking money for a quick fix will go bare for a few pounds more. This is an ideal bridging group for spread of infection into the heterosexual community.

There is also the possibility of secret intravenous drug

abusers having normal relationships with non-users. They may be infected, but asymptomatic and with no knowledge of the danger they pose. Even an ex-addict may be infected, having changed their lifestyle, and may infect other people in the course of later relationships.

Intravenous drug abusers pose the greatest threat for heterosexual spread into society at large. To date there has been little evidence of this in Ireland, but we must heed the warnings from elsewhere, as in the United States, where heterosexual transmission of AIDS is mostly from drug users. In women it has the additional potential to infect their offspring.

BABIES OF INTRAVENOUS DRUG ABUSERS
Number tested: 34 — HIVab+ 23 — 68%

All the known cases of HIVab+ babies in Ireland were infected before birth by their mothers. In at least one case several HIVab+ children were born to one mother before she was sterilised. Two children have progressed to AIDS. Some are awaiting repeat antibody testing to find out if they really are infected after clearance of their maternal antibodies. (It takes about six months for newborn babies to lose the antibodies they have got from their mothers, and so it is only after this time that we can find out if they have antibodies of their own.) Dublin has the second largest incidence of paediatric HIV infection in Europe and the problem is the subject of a special study funded by the EEC.

It is noteworthy that of eighty-four known female HIV-infected intravenous drug abusers that thirty-four of them, or 40 per cent, managed to get pregnant in the short period that we have had the HIVab test available for surveillance. One wonders how many infected girls there are in the community, how many of them are pregnant or have had their babies without detection. As the early signs of HIV infection in the newborn child may be relatively non-specific, this is entirely possible. One wonders about the nature of the care, counselling and follow-up that gives a failure rate of 40 per cent in a short period of time and that has allowed thirty-four new HIV-infected cases to be conceived.

There is a high probability of HIV-infected babies becoming very sick over the first two to three years of their life. Whilst many intravenous drug abusers make good, caring mothers, there are some that cannot cope, even with healthy children. Too often these children will be destined to be taken into institutional care or into the care of local authorities and they may become 'AIDS orphans' if their parents die of their infection. The prospects for adoption and fostering may be remote for these children, and they face the potential of life-long institutional care. Adequate identification of those at risk, counselling and follow-up with proper contraceptive measures could prevent a lot of this human misery.

HOMOSEXUALS/BISEXUALS
Number tested: 1080 — HIVab+ 58 — 5.4%

This is the group that took the first toll of AIDS in the western world and with whom the disease was most associated, but not so in Ireland. When the HIVab test was first available in Ireland in early 1985, a substantial proportion of those coming for testing at STD clinics were found to be positive, in the order of 25 per cent in one area. However, it soon became clear that this was the result of bias: those with the greatest fear or who had some symptoms suggestive of HIV infection came for testing first. Soon the rate dropped to the order of 12-14 per cent, where it remained for some time. Because of fears regarding confidentiality, and the implications that a positive result would hamper future insurance, mortgage and job prospects as well as anxiety over the ability to cope with a positive result, the Gay Health Action Group actively discouraged the test. We are now probably seeing an opposite bias towards a falsely low HIVab+ rate, as many of the attenders are the 'worried well' with no real apparent risk of contracting the infection, but with considerable anxiety often induced by publicity and health education campaigns.

In areas of high prevalence, such as London, Manhattan and the west coast of America, the assumption is almost made that people in the high-risk groups are positive, and results show that 32 per cent of homosexual men attending a central London

STD clinic are HIVab+ and as high as 60 per cent in some United States cities. These figures are biased and vary substantially from area to area. In central London, adjacent areas can vary widely with other clinics reporting only a 12 per cent positivity rate in their homosexual population. Gay patients may choose to attend a clinic where they know they will be well received and looked after, and this introduces a bias to the rates of infection reported. Individual cases tend to cluster in core groups and locations and frequently there may be a chain of contact within these groups. It is addressing these core groups that will bring most cost-effective benefit in containing the infection.

Outside the high prevalence areas, such as metropolitan London, the HIVab+ rate falls off substantially and for instance the English provincial cities have only had prevalence in the order of 2-10 per cent. They have only had sporadic cases of AIDS so far. Dublin would fit in with this pattern, but with a smaller number of known HIVab+ cases. It is unusual in having an apparent fall in the number of cases of homosexually acquired AIDS in the past two years.

HAEMOPHILIACS
Number tested: 510 — HIVab+ 107 — 21%

These patients were infected by contaminated Factor VIII prepared from large donor pools in the United States. Most of the infection occurred in the early 1980s and once the virus was isolated and identified, the problem was tackled by screening blood donors and by heating the Factor VIII to a level that kills the virus without inactivating the clotting factor. For this reason we do not expect any new cases in this group.

The chances of infection depend upon the severity of the haemophilia. Almost 70 per cent of those with severe haemophilia type A, requiring large amounts of Factor VIII, are infected, whilst only 15 per cent with mild haemophilia type A are infected. Twenty per cent of severe haemophilia B are infected and none with mild haemophilia B.

The majority of haemophiliacs at risk, especially those with a high requirement for Factor VIII, have been tested. The majority of patients are under the care of the National Haemophilia Treatment Centre.

The burden of haemophilia is enough for any person to have to bear. Factor VIII has revolutionised the lives of haemophiliacs and allows them to lead full and relatively normal lives. Despite the risk of HIV infection, most would say that they would prefer to use Factor VIII and take the risk, as life would be limited and unbearable without it. Fortunately that risk has now been almost totally removed, but we are left with a substantial group of people who have to carry the additional burden of HIV infection as well as haemophilia, people who were infected before screening was introduced.

Some of these are children attending school. There is no risk to other children at school, unless one is to consider sex and intravenous drug abuse in the older child, though obviously practices such as 'blood brotherhood' are to be avoided and basic hygiene observed. There are no reports of parents of other children over-reacting to the presence of an antibody positive haemophiliac child in Irish schools, though it has happened in other countries, and of course there is always the danger of these children being stigmatised by the often cruel practices of childhood.

Adult haemophiliacs face the same problem of stigma in society and the tiresome responsibility to follow safe sex guidelines. This can pose considerable strain on a person, both in adolescence and within a relationship or marriage. Many haemophiliacs have decided against having children anyway for fear that they might be haemophiliacs, and this infection adds an even more potent argument for this. Spouses stand an approximate 10 per cent chance of becoming infected, but happily none of those tested so far in Ireland have done so to date.

NON-CATEGORISED
Number tested: 5201 — HIVab+ 25 — 0.004%

Most of these were non-categorised because of incomplete data on their request form but were probably in the intravenous drug abuse group. Two of the cases represented a couple that were from Central Africa.

What is most noteworthy about this group is the enormous number who have been tested and found to be free from infection. Most of these constitute the 'worried well' who had some episode or activity that made them anxious to be checked. Many had had prostitute contact either here or abroad, but none have been infected as yet. Prostitute contact is cited as a factor in the 'no known risk' group for AIDS in the United States.

Many of this group attended because of media publicity and public health education campaigns about AIDS, both here and abroad. The experience that none of these have been positive mirrors that in England and raises the question whether this is the best way to spend our scarce resources. However, other sexually transmitted diseases were found in many of these people.

In addition to these groups all blood donations in this country are tested, and so far out of over 200,000 tested, only four have been found to be positive. This positivity rate is less than in Britain.

GROUPS HIVab NEGATIVE TO 30/9/86

NUMBER	TESTED
CONTACTS OF HAEMOPHILIACS	28
NEEDLE-STICK INJURY	45
TRANSFUSION RECIPIENTS	26
ORGAN DONORS	25
VISA APPLICANTS*	267

*People applying for visas to visit Saudi Arabia or Japan are required to undergo an HIVab test

The fact that no haemophiliac contacts have become infected points to the efficacy of good counselling and prevention through safe sex practices and use of condoms. The absence of infection through needle-stick injury reflects results obtained from other studies. We have had no transfusion recipients infected either now or prior to the introduction of routine donor testing, which implies a low general prevalence of the infection in Ireland. Nor have any of the visa applicants been found to be infected.

AIDS IN NORTHERN IRELAND
Dr Raymond Maw

To the end of March 1987 there had been two definite cases of AIDS diagnosed for the first time in Northern Ireland. Both cases had occurred in homosexual males who were natives of Northern Ireland but were domiciled outside of Ireland and had undoubtedly acquired their infection outside. Neither patient had any sexual contact in Northern Ireland, but one Dublin contact was subsequently shown to have a positive blood test. One of these patients died of *Pneumocystis carinii* pneumonia in 1985 and the other is still alive. One possible case has been diagnosed retrospectively in a patient who died in the Royal Victoria Hospital in 1984. This patient had an undiagnosed pyrexial illness and came from an area where AIDS is endemic. He gave a history of heterosexual contact only and a blood test carried out on stored serum has been shown to be positive. One other case was incorrectly diagnosed as AIDS but this has subsequently been changed to ARC. This man was a heterosexual with a history of sexual intercourse with prostitutes in South America and he had had a blood transfusion in the United States in the early 1980s.

In addition to these cases there have been eleven positive blood tests from the Genito-Urinary Medicine Department in Belfast, nine in homosexual patients and two in bisexuals. Of these eleven patients, five were from outside Ireland. None were long-term residents in Northern Ireland, but three had had sexual contact with gay partners in Northern Ireland, thus possibly introducing the virus into the community. The six Northern Ireland residents, with the exception of one, had histories of sexual contact in London and the United States. The one without such a history acquired the infection from his partner who had recently returned from London.

This pattern of infected persons coming in from abroad and having sexual contact with a community unexposed to the infection is precisely the pattern that could be forecast for establishing a disease such as HIV infection in a community. It is, of course, a very short step from this phase to the establishment of endemic infection in the community, so that avoidance of sexual contact with 'outsiders' is no longer an effective way of preventing spread of infection. This point needs to be clearly recognised to avoid a false sense of security which some gay males may have that sex with 'locals' is still safe.

Two heterosexual men have been identified as positive, one of whom is not a resident of Northern Ireland. Their risk factors were sexual intercourse in Central Africa in one case and in the other intercourse with a prostitute in Amsterdam. No women have been identified as positive in Northern Ireland, nor have any infants been positive.

The number of haemophiliac patients identified as being infected is sixteen which is 16.5 per cent of the haemophiliacs in Northern Ireland treated with Factor VIII concentrate. This is the smallest percentage for any country in Europe for this group, becasue it happened that the Factor VIII used in Northern Ireland was drawn from predominantly European sources in the past rather than from predominantly American sources. None of the haemophiliacs have developed AIDS nor have any of their sexual contacts had a positive blood test.

All blood donors are now asked to sign a declaration that they consent to their blood being tested for HIV infection and since October 1985 in excess of 80,000 donations have been tested. Two tests were positive and both of these patients were referred to the Genito-Urinary Medicine Department and their cases have been included in the data given on that clinic.

Unlike the situation in Dublin, there is a very small number of intravenous drug abusers in Belfast. This may be partially because the paramilitary organisations actively discourage drug abuse in their areas of operation, but this cannot be a full explanation as their spheres of influence are mostly confined to working-class areas and intravenous drug abuse is not confined to this social group. Of the small number of known intravenous drug abusers tested, none have been positive for HIV infection.

The recent advertising campaign on AIDS by the UK government has undoubtedly raised public awareness of this problem. Unfortunately such an advertising campaign cannot avoid arousing anxieties in many people and this has certainly been reflected in the pattern of requests for HIV testing at the Genito-Urinary Medicine Department and from other medical practitioners. Up to December 1986 just over two hundred had been tested in the Genito-Urinary Medicine Department in Belfast, the large majority of whom were gay men. Between January and March 1987 when the campaign was at its peak, 275 were tested of whom 234 were heterosexuals, most of whom had no known risk factors. Many of these people exhibited severe anxiety symptoms requiring prolonged counselling. This by-product of public education on AIDS needs to be clearly recognised by governments, both in designing future campaigns and in providing a service to cope with such problems.

A vigorous response by the health boards in the province and voluntary organisations is aimed at providing accurate information and adequate services to meet the demands that may be made on them. The four health boards have developed strategies for dealing with AIDS. The largest board, the Eastern Health and Social Services Board, has set up an AIDS steering group to implement its policy document. The major task as perceived by this group is preventive education of the public with specific emphasis on health-care personnel and young people. A group has been established to devise education packages for schools and it is hoped that these will be acceptable to all secondary schools in the province. Other points of note in the board's policy are the provision of free condoms at the Genito-Urinary Medicine Department and family planning clinics. Sales of condoms from chemists have risen dramatically in early 1987. The need to identify intravenous drug abusers and provide them with clean needles and syringes to prevent a spread of infection has been clearly recognised. The board has also issued a statement that no person in its employment will lose their job if found to be positive.

The lead for the voluntary organisations' response to AIDS was given by the Carafriend association. This is the local gay voluntary body, which in the past has established a helpline and befriending network for gays in Northern Ireland. Carafriend has actively campaigned among its members for the adoption of safe sex practices and can be seen to have given a responsible lead to their community. In addition to this, Carafriend members were responsible for setting up the AIDS helpline in Belfast which is manned by heterosexual and homosexual volunteers three nights a week. The helpline is now totally independent of Carafriend and is a service for the whole community. This service provides a telephone line whereby people who are worried can speak to trained personnel about their worries and ask for advice, which may only need to be reassurance in many cases, but in other cases referral to other agencies is advised or a meeting with one of the volunteers for further counselling and advice. This has proved an invaluable service and it receives funding from the Northern Ireland Department of Health and Social Services.

The public response to AIDS in Northern Ireland cannot yet be accurately assessed. A number of initiatives trying to measure attitudes and knowledge about AIDS have been carried out but no results are yet available. No fall in the incidence of common sexually transmitted diseases has been observed among the heterosexual attenders at the Genito-Urinary Medicine Department, but there has been a definite fall in the number of cases of infection in gay men and a marked change in sexual behaviour has been reported by this group.

Northern Ireland could be described as a society on the brink of having a serious problem with AIDS. The situation is certainly more hopeful than for other western communities if the lessons already learnt can be taken on board by the sexually active community, both heterosexual and homosexual.

There has been a substantial rise over the past ten years in incidents of other sexually transmitted diseases, such as genital warts and non-specific urethritis. That rise parallels that seen in the rest of the United Kingdom, although the incidence per hundred thousand of population lags behind in Northern Ireland by approximately five years. On this basis we would expect AIDS to be a major health-care problem in the next few years unless a major change in sexual behaviour is seen to occur in the immediate future.

STRATEGY AND PREVENTION

Although the actual number of cases of AIDS has been small to date in Ireland, the potential for spread is immense, particularly when one looks at the number of people infected with the virus both here and abroad. We have a particular risk in Ireland with a high number of intravenous drug abusers infected, who in the United States have accounted for most of the heterosexual transmission of AIDS as well as the problem of infection in the newborn.

It was difficult to develop a cogent strategy in the early days of the epidemic as initially one did not know what one was dealing with. It was important to develop an adequate and reliable reporting system so that one could follow the epidemic. We are left with the main problem of dealing with the infection in the homosexual and intravenous drug abusing risk groups, and prevention in the general public who would often not consider themselves to be at risk.

The current strategy in most countries is to adopt a public health information campaign aimed at the general population, and one has just been launched at time of going to press. At this stage it is questionable whether this is the best way to expend our very scarce resources. The effect of the media campaign in Great Britain was that clinic attendances increased by a factor of two to four times, but the number of new cases of HIVab+ patients found was very small. The clinics had no additional staff or resources to face this influx of people, so it is unlikely that they were able to provide the kind of counselling people coming looking for this test should have. However, the public was certainly forced to face AIDS infection as an issue of everyday life which ordinary people may have to confront personally if they have been exposed to any risks. Before the campaign, there was evidence that people knew a great deal about AIDS, but only a proportion were prepared to alter their habits, especially when it came to reducing the number of sex partners and using condoms in the younger age groups. Following the campaign there has been an increased awareness of these factors, but not of a substantial amount. The campaign circus has left town, but what is left behind to continue to drive home and reinforce the message?

Surveys show that we in Ireland are already quite knowledgeable about AIDS, and that this awareness is not confined to the multi-channel television areas on the east coast. Most people know how AIDS is transmitted, and a surprisingly small percentage thinks that it can be caught by social contact. Very few people were in favour of segragating HIV-infected people, making AIDS a notifiable disease or compulsory blood-testing. It appears that the media have already done a good job in informing the public about this disease and have done so at surprisingly little cost to the tax payer. (See *Sunday World* article — details in bibliography.)

At this stage of the evolution of the problem we need to develop a strategy. The strategy should be simple and have attainable aims: containment and care.

Containment
Containment involves reduction in the spread of the disease. Apart from the personal consequences and risk of spread in society, each case of AIDS is estimated to cost in the region of £20,000—£40,000 to care for; even if we only reduce the cases of AIDS by 50 per cent, the pay-off in terms of alleviation of personal suffering and cost to the health services and society

as a whole is immense. Containment programmes must be aimed at the specific risk groups where the prevalence of infection is highest and the public in general help them to recognise and avoid risk activities.

As elsewhere, we in Ireland have little information on the **homosexual population** in Ireland. People's sexuality is after all a private concern and intrusion is actively guarded against and resented. In Ireland homosexual practices remain a criminal offence and many gays are driven to secrecy. The practice is condemned by the church and many homosexuals are fearful of the attitude of their family and friends.

Those who have most to fear are the covert or secret gays who are afraid to make any permanent relationships, so often make casual contacts in parks or on the quays. They may meet a substantial number of partners in a year. Bisexuals are often married and are also secretive in their habits and fear that a permanent gay relationship may break up their marriage. But casual relationships put their own lives and the lives of their spouses and unborn children at risk.

Many male homosexuals probably lead a very repressed and covert life in Ireland, some turning to marriage to conceal their orientation, but over the past ten to fifteen years an era of openness and awareness has developed, especially in Dublin and Cork, where gay centres have become established and gay rights have found expression both socially and politically. This has encouraged many to come out and declare their orientation, and this new mood of openness has provided an infrastructure for informing gay men about the dangers of infection. Out of the gay organisations the Gay Health Action Group was formed. This group, on its own initiative and with little or no funding, set about informing people, organising lectures, producing leaflets, providing a telephone helpline service and set up an HIVab+ counselling group. This occurred years before anybody else saw the need. They have provided a caring service to the community at large, on a voluntary basis, and at no cost to the health services. They have been rewarded with an apparent low HIVab+ rate and a reduction in the rate of AIDS cases in this group since 1985.

In the United States, the doubling time of the epidemic has

gone from six months to thirteen months among homosexuals, so it seems that gay health initiatives are working. Behavioural practices have changed dramatically with well-documented evidence and reduction in the number of partners and avoidance of anal intercourse. This has been achieved through self-help groups and groups that have arisen out of the gay community and that relate to the gay community. Their success points to the necessity and efficiency of providing services through existing community structures and personnel who relate to the particular group and who are seen as credible to that group. It would seem sensible and economic to build upon the existing infrastructure and to support it.

Though most homosexuals have acted responsibly since the discovery of how AIDS is transmitted, there remains a core group of men who continue to make casual sexual contacts and who are not accessible or amenable to health education measures. Such people are a risk to the community, and bisexuals especially may form a bridging group to the heterosexual community, picking up the infection from homosexual partners and passing it on to their wives or other women partners.

The **intravenous drug abusing community** is more of a challenge. Intravenous drug abusers tend to come from a more deprived section of society and their addictive habits alienate them from society. Their horizon may be limited to the next fix. Although there is a camaraderie among them it is not organised to any positive ends and is mainly concerned with the availability of drugs. Withdrawal from the drugs is very hard, and it is commonplace to fall back into the habit. Containment and reduction of the infection in this group must be achieved as the most urgent priority. In the United States, there is alarm that the rise in the intravenous drug abusing related cases has continued unabated. In Europe between 30 and 70 per cent of intravenous drug abusers in southern Spain, southern France and Italy have been reported to be infected, and data shows that the rise in infection rates can be explosive once it enters the community. This group poses a great risk to society in general. In the United States heterosexual transmission of the infection is mostly from drug users. It is the main route of the infection to prostitutes, who pose a risk to society as a whole if they do not use condoms. The spread of HIV infection in drug users will be the main source for any future heterosexual epidemic in the western world, and we in Ireland may be particularly vulnerable to this. Not only does this group cause spread by heterosexual transmission but many girls and young women become pregnant and bear infected children. In Ireland there are eighty-four known infected females, of whom 40 per cent became pregnant and had children in a short period of time. Seventy per cent of their babies were infected.

We do not have a great deal in the way of services to cope with the drug addiction problem in this country, let alone the possibility of an AIDS epidemic. The National Drugs Advisory and Treatment Centre at Jervis Street Hospital has a small detoxification department and inadequate out-patient services. Few general medical practitioners are in a position to help, both because of lack of training and expertise in this field and because of the fierce manipulative pressures that intravenous drug abusers can impose. Voluntary projects, like Coolmine and Ana-Liffey, have helped enormously and the church has been active both in these projects and in the community. But this is not enough. If we are to contain the problem we must invest heavily in services for the core groups.

We must face the primary problem of drug abuse. In particular we must face the pushers who like parasites flourish on the misery and degradation of others. We must face the question of social, moral and economic deprivation in the community found to be most affected by the problem. We must help parents to deal with large families, and target those families with a history of addiction to other substances, such as alcohol and cigarettes, which may be more socially acceptable but provide a pointer for an increased potential of drug abuse. We must provide a safety net for the children where the parents cannot cope and where community relationships have broken down and neighbours cannot offer support. We must fight apathy and acceptance, and support community projects on the ground. We need more counsellors in the community who can give addicts and those at risk somewhere to turn to other than the pusher. There is a group of people emerging from rehabilitation programmes, such as Coolmine, who may be sufficiently strong and resourceful to go back into the abusing community and use their personal knowledge and experience to help others fight their addiction, as well as working with those in danger of addiction.

General health education is likely to go well over the heads of the intravenous drug abusers who may see themselves as apart and alienated anyway. The question of literacy in this population has to be addressed. Many start abusing drugs in late childhood and early teens, and they must be addressed in childhood. Prevention and education programmes must be not only directly aimed at these core groups, but also at their friends, families, teachers and neighbours, so that the full horrors of drug abuse become known and so that support is provided for the vulnerable and pushers are treated with the contempt they deserve.

In some countries sterile needles are supplied to addicts in an effort to combat the spread of AIDS infection by preventing sharing of needles but such schemes, though they sometimes seem to work, are open to abuse, and a clean needle programme does nothing to reduce the basic problem — drug abuse.

Containment among drug addicts also means the prevention of conception as there is a 70 per cent chance of an infected mother having an infected baby, with a 50 per cent progression rate to AIDS both in the mother and in the newborn. It is not pleasant to be told that you should not conceive, especially if you are a young girl longing for the role of motherhood, so counselling and follow-up with reinforcement of the message are necessary. Of course it is also necessary to provide adequate and reliable contraception.

Containment in the **general population** can be achieved through informing people how the infection is contracted and what the risk activities are. This is being achieved to a considerable extent, but the message needs to be constantly reinforced and public awareness needs to be kept high. Young people are most at risk and in youngsters the infection has a longer time to be present and to progress perhaps to full AIDS.

We must face the fact that while we may seek to change human nature, we are unlikely to succeed, but if we are successful in modifying it to the extent that most people will avoid risk activities it should be possible to prevent a large number of cases.

Health education from an early age is an important preventive measure. The United States Surgeon General, R. Everett Koop, was well known as a conservative in regard to health education in schools, but now he states that education about AIDS must start at the earliest possible level. This is common sense as children may start to abuse drugs from the age of nine or ten and we are beginning to see some pre-teen pregnancies. Sex education in schools should inform children of the facts and should emphasise that one has to have a responsibility in sexuality, both to oneself and to one's partner.

Care

As a society we have set ourselves a model of caring for those less fortunate who are in poorer health than ourselves, and this care and compassion is central to our whole moral and ethical ethos.

Caring for people with HIV infection or AIDS has put this to the test for some people. Community care services, particularly primary medical care, offer an open-access and 'unlabelled' service with continuity of care. This is only possible if the individuals providing the service are knowledgeable about AIDS and are prepared to deal with the problem and the people. Above all they must be prepared to observe the basic rules of dealing with AIDS, the three Cs: Consent, Confidentiality and Counselling. If they cannot do this, they should recognise it in themselves and be kind enough to refer the person to another who can. Compassion is the basic minimum that is expected.

Primary care in the community involves not only the general practitioner, but the entire team and resources of the community care services in continuing care of the patient and his or her family. Some patients are prisoners, and pose special problems of their own with the additional pressures of isolation and loss of contact from society and relatives. Other primary contacts will be made in casualty departments, emergency admissions to hospitals and in family planning clinics, which are often seen as 'a good place to take one's genitals to'.

To achieve the aim of containment, provision of care is a basic necessity. One can only expect the high-risk groups to respond to exhortations if they are offered a caring and supportive service on the ground. This will necessitate the provision of people who are skilled and knowledgeable, particularly in the core 'at-risk' populations. Education and training courses will be required for these personnel and also for primary care doctors.

Not all primary health-care providers are suited, either temperamentally or organisationally, to care for HIV-infected people. Some may be able to care for the sexually acquired infections but may not be able to cope with the pressures and manipulations of the intravenous drug abusers. Special knowledge and full support from other community and hospital services are required with a good basic knowledge of sexually transmitted diseases and the problems of intravenous drug abusers. Professionalism is being firm, in control, and there is no place for addiction management in primary care, unless one has a recognised and supported expertise in this area.

Secondary care of HIV infection and AIDS is based in the STD clinics and the drug dependency units in Ireland and some specialised units in hospitals. In Ireland it is more of an evolving system than any structured scheme. HIV-related cases require counselling either to deal with an infection or to ensure that they do not acquire an infection. It is essential that the STD service is augmented and supported to provide care and counselling for HIV-related problems if there is to be any hope of containing this epidemic. The drug treatment unit finds itself in a similar position and failure to answer the needs of these services will result in more extensive spread within the core groups and a greater risk of spread into the community at large.

Tertiary care of HIV infection takes place at specialised units in hospitals which are required for the diagnosis of some of the opportunistic infections. Also the haemophiliac cases are handled through the haemophiliac units. There has been a close working relationship between the staff in the haemophiliac units and their patients. HIV infection has added to the burden of work carried out in these units and also to the personal strain that results from involvement with these tragic cases.

It is planned that every hospital should be able to look after HIV-infected and AIDS cases. However, practice makes perfect and some units will emerge which will have developed a special expertise in dealing with this problem.

In San Francisco, where the widest experience exists in dealing with AIDS, the strategy is to try and reduce hospitalisation as much as possible and then strive for as normal a life as possible. This is done through community care services and hostels or hospices for those who are unable to look after themselves. They have evolved the 'buddy' system where each AIDS patient is paired with a volunteer who undertakes to look after them for the duration of their disease. The programmes have been very successful both on a personal and institutional level. It is likely that they will be emulated elsewhere.

To plan an effective strategy one needs to have an idea of the size and distribution of the at-risk groups. We urgently need some good demographic studies to guide us how to best use our resources to target the at-risk groups, and we need to involve the groups in doing so.

The Gay Health Action Group and more recently the Catholic Social Service Conference Task Force on AIDS have taken the initiative. It is likely that the immense resources of the church will be used to care for infected and ill people. We are still waiting for our public health service, with a budget in excess of a billion pounds a year, to spend a few thousand pounds to help those with problems and to provide the basic infrastructure necessary to care for the core groups affected — STD clinics and drug treatment centres.

CHAPTER 4

INTRAVENOUS DRUG ABUSE AND AIDS

By Fr Paul Lavelle

During the summer of 1986 I met Peter, aged twenty-four, at a Narcotics Anonymous meeting. Peter had AIDS. He was down and extremely angry. He said there were no supports available to him in Ireland, and he regretted that he wasn't gay because at least the gay community supports members of their own group who have AIDS-related problems. This encounter with Peter had an influence on me and I suddenly realised the potentially serious situation which would develop, particularly in Dublin, over the next few years with intravenous drug abusers.

INCREASE IN DRUG ABUSE IN DUBLIN

In June 1982, Dr Geoffrey Dean, director of the Medico-Social Research Board, investigated reports of an increase of heroin misuse in Dublin during the previous twelve months. Until the spring of 1981 there had apparently been very little misuse of heroin in the Republic, but at that time a heroin epidemic began in Dublin, probably sparked off by the huge influx of heroin onto the world market consequent on the Iranian revolution in late 1980.

In the winter of 1982/3, an investigation of heroin misuse in a north central Dublin area was carried out. It showed that in the area studied, eighty-eight young people (that is 10 per cent of the fifteen-to-twenty-four-year-olds) were using heroin of whom two were experimenters, four were using it two or

92

three times a week and eighty-two at least once daily. In 1983 the National Drugs Advisory and Treatment Centre in Jervis Street Hospital in Dublin treated 1500 people. January 1984 showed a 45 per cent increase over January 1983. About 80 per cent of those treated were opiate users, heroin being the main drug of choice. It is estimated that there are approximately 3000 heroin users in the Dublin area.

Misuse was mainly by young people. A good deal of crime was associated with this misuse since purchase of the needed heroin commonly called for the expenditure of £100 a day for each user. At that time there was an alarming increase in the number of persons charged with the possession of opiates and an increase in the number of drug users being committed to prison.

Recently a further report gathering information on seventy-four of the original eighty-eight heroin users was compiled. At the time of re-interview (1985/6) twenty-two were still on heroin, twenty-three in prison, eleven attending methadone maintenance programmes and eighteen were heroin-free. Seventy-six per cent of the sample were under twenty-five years, with the majority single or separated. The single or separated parents had a total of sixty children. Since the time of initial interview, sixty-nine respondents had attempted to give up heroin, primarily through a detoxification programme, fifty-five had attended hospital for drug related conditions, sixty-six had been unemployed and forty-nine had served prison sentences. At that time it was not ascertained what the position was regarding the HIV virus but an accurate figure would suggest there are about 22 per cent of that group with the antibodies.

Large quantities of heroin are available on the international market and Ireland is a target country for international traffickers. It is easily smuggled and is a lucrative commodity. Furthermore, it is extremely addictive and expensive. Many habitual users become pushers and this creates more addicts, so increasing the demand. Also, more addicts are forced to turn to crime to pay for their addiction and we have witnessed an escalating crime problem in recent years in Ireland. The rewards for heroin smuggling are enormous: a spoonful is worth about £900. In the late 1970s and early 1980s organised crime became involved in drugs in Dublin and certain criminal families controlled a major section of the Irish market.

Over the past few years the heroin problem has flourished in Dublin's inner city, in areas stricken by poverty, unemployment, illiteracy, poor housing and broken families. The main problem with heroin abuse is the enormous psychological dependency, rather than the physical dependency, it creates. However, the damage to the body also is enormous: hepatitis, abscesses, gangrene and now the HIV. Some take drugs to bring relief from boredom and depression or for kicks. They are lonely and insecure and see this as a way out. However, the fundamental and most important factor is the availability of the drugs.

WHO IS ABUSING DRUGS?

There is no area of Dublin that has not got some of its young people in attendance at the Jervis Street treatment centre. Over the past few years, the problem was more serious in the socially and educationally under-privileged inner-city areas, but there is now increasing evidence that drug abuse has become more prevalent in middle-class areas.

The average age of first contact with drugs is seventeen. Alarmingly it usually takes two to four years before the problem of drug abuse is recognised in the person. Also, there is generally a three-year gap between first contact with hard drugs and seeking help in treatment centres. The typical user seeking treatment is twenty-one years of age, has been using drugs for four years, is mainlining heroin, has been in trouble with the law and is unemployed. There is usually a background of stress in the family — heavy drinking by a parent or the illness, death or separation of a parent. The user normally was unhappy at school and dropped out early. Addicts do not set out to become addicted: they firmly believe that addiction only happens to others. When addicted to a drug it becomes the driving force in their lives and they will do anything to acquire it. Drug addicts lose all self-esteem and their moral standards decline. They will lie, be dishonest and will manipulate anyone, especially those closest to them, to get drugs.

Most drug users have enormous financial, emotional, social and family problems. They are a difficult group to deal with because of their aggressiveness, deceptiveness and ability to manipulate, but they are a compassionate group, who have known what it is to suffer over the years, rely on their emotions rather than their intellect — because it has never been developed — are good neighbours, generous to a fault, good-humoured and humble.

THE HIV

In February 1987 it was confirmed that 360 intravenous drug abusers had tested positive to the HIV virus. Dr Zachary Johnson of the Eastern Health Board suggests that there are almost certainly about 1600 people in Ireland carrying antibodies to the HIV. It is known that about 60 per cent of the total tested from the higher risk groups are from the intravenous drug abuser population. Therefore we can assume that there are about 960 intravenous drug users who presently carry the virus, many of whom will go on to develop AIDS and who, while appearing healthy, are capable of infecting others through needle-sharing or sexual contact. I have no doubt that this group is the most at risk and will be the group to transmit the virus and spread it into the heterosexual population.

It is more important now to contain the spread of AIDS even than to deal with the drug abuse problem. This is also the conclusion of the Scottish committee on HIV infection and intravenous drug use who studied the problem in Edinburgh,which in many ways is similar to the Irish situation. Drug abuse messes up your life, but AIDS kills — it kills drug addicts, their sexual partners and their unborn children. There are twenty-two babies in this country at present, children of intravenous drug users, who are antibody positive.

Intravenous drug users must be informed and counselled about the risks they undertake in continuing their use. They must also be offered support and assistance in trying to make themselves drug-free. They must be counselled not to inject drugs, but if they do then they must be counselled to take precautions and to use clean needles.

STRATEGIES

1. Health education: A national educational campaign, explicit, giving information on the transmission of this virus, is essential. However, it is unlikely to reach the drug-using population. What is essential amongst this group is a change in behaviour: information in itself is unlikely to do this. What is needed is direct one-to-one contact, which can be done by outreach workers within the community. There is evidence that counselling will help some to change behaviour.

2. Consideration of provision of sterile equipment: Pilot schemes have now been introduced in twelve centres in the United Kingdom. Needle-exchange is only part of an overall programme. Although the provision of clean needles seems to condone drug use, to be inconsistent with the aims of drug abstinence programmes and to undermine the work of health-care workers, there are arguments in favour of wider availability of clean syringes. There is no evidence that increased availability leads to increased use of drugs and distribution has the advantage of bringing users into contact with treatment centres and counsellors. For some this may be the first step in a treatment programme. And a clean syringe helps others who are at risk from infection — innocent sexual partners and children.

3. Substitute prescribing (methadone maintenance): This is also controversial, and many experts hold different views. There is no doubt that some users could be persuaded to give up injecting drugs as a first step before becoming drug-free. This strategy could be considered for those whom it is judged it would assist in reducing or stopping injecting. It would also be a means of maintaining contact with drug users.

4. Extension of existing services: If we are to address the problem of AIDS, it is essential to address the problems of drug misuse. Long-term medical care and social care, as well as counselling, need to be provided.

The intravenous drug using group will be the most difficult to target and any health education campaign which does not make one-to-one contact will, I believe, fail. They are the group most likely to transmit the virus to the heterosexual community and are the most difficult group in terms of trying to modify behaviour.

THE MORAL ISSUES

There are difficult moral issues involved in the prevention of the spread of the HIV. Condoms and free needles and syringes for drug addicts will reduce but not remove the dangers of HIV infection or the spread of the virus. The message should be: Don't do drugs, but if you are going to, then don't share the equipment and make sure that it is sterile.

For many people, especially for Catholics, the use of condoms is morally wrong, but there is a theological opinion that the use of condoms in marriage can be justified where the intention is not to prevent conception but to prevent spread of an infection. The intention re-defines the use of a condom in marital intercourse: because there is no contraceptive intent it is not a contraceptive act.

The church's view is that sexual relationships outside of marriage are morally wrong. I would ask if homosexual activity, adultery or fornication are any more sinful or wrong if protection is taken against transmitting a deadly disease. It is difficult to see how this could be. If a person is engaging in such sexual activity it would appear to be more responsible to use a condom: indeed it would appear to be irresponsible not to where there is a danger of infecting another person. So our message in this case is: Don't do sex outside of marriage. But if you don't accept the Christian teaching and are sexually active then use a condom to help prevent the risk of infection. (However, condoms are not foolproof, and it would be misleading to give people a false sense of security about their use.)

AIDS AND THE WRATH OF GOD

AIDS is God's wrath only if cancer, diabetes, heart disease or other diseases people suffer from are all signs of God's wrath as well. God does not punish through disease. God's love and grace is total and unconditional.

When a person with leprosy, who not alone had a physical

disease but was a social outcast as well, approached Jesus, he asked if he wanted to accept and heal him. Jesus's immediate response was ' Of course I want to — be cured' (Mark 1.41). Through the New Testament teachings of Jesus we learn that the link between sin and disease is broken and the link between forgiveness and love is realised.

It is important to remember that among those who will suffer from AIDS will be spouses and children, who have unwittingly contracted the virus. The God of the new convenant does not wish to wipe out drug addicts, babies of mothers who abuse drugs, homosexuals and, in some strange way, clumsily kill haemophiliacs in the process. AIDS is an illness, not a sin.

THE CHURCH RESPONSE
In January 1987, the Catholic bishops of Ireland realised that we could be on the edge of an epidemic of AIDS in Ireland. They called in the first place for a compassionate and caring attitude towards those with the HIV and with AIDS. Accepting the need to prevent the spread of the disease, they stated that it would be sad if the response to this major threat were to be reduced simply to a debate about free needles or easy availability of condoms. They called for a more active programme of education towards the prevention of drug abuse and warned of the great dangers posed by the abuse of sex — 'the precious gift of sexual love is reserved in its full expression for the life-long, life-giving, exclusive union of two people in marriage'.

In March 1987 a national task force was set up at the bishops' request by the Catholic Social Service Conference with District Justice Julian Hussey as chairperson and myself as full-time pastoral care co-ordinator. This group was allocated an initial budget of £20,000. The task force will use whatever resources the church has in caring for those who are antibody positive or have AIDS. It is hoped also to use all the educational resources at its disposal. In concluding, the bishops said, ' We trust that the establishment of the new task force will mark the beginning of a response from the Irish church which will be generous, practical and compassionate.'

Section III

CHAPTER 5

COUNSELLING AND ADVICE

In dealing with an infection for which there is no known cure and no vaccination, with a potential to progress to AIDS which carries a prognosis as bad as the worst cancer, our only weapons are prevention through knowledge and care through support. Faced with such a potential prospect, people who are anxious or at risk have sometimes an overwhelming anxiety and need counselling. They are usually very well informed about the disease and expect those who advise them to be equally well informed. Anybody can provide support and counselling, provided they have the knowledge of the disease and have the personal strength to see people through their crisis. Many people coming for advice or testing in Ireland are the 'worried well' at present and we can be happy to advise them that they are very unlikely to be infected or, following testing, that they are not infected.

Doctors and counsellors working in areas of higher prevalence find it difficult not to become involved in the tragedy of young people dying from an infectious disease, with little to offer them apart from themselves as support. This is an experience unknown to the last two generations of doctors.

RISK OF INFECTION

Angst, fear and anguish are the hallmarks of AIDS. Many people are anxious regarding the risk of contracting the infection from what we would term 'non-risk activities'. Most people really know that it would be extremely unlikely for them to have contracted an infection, but are merely seeking a further personal reassurance for themselves. In fact it is quite hard to contract this infection: it needs to be directly inoculated from one person to another. Yet AIDS helplines are bombarded with enquiries: Can you get AIDS from a swimming pool? Is it safe to share cutlery and eating utensils? I kissed a man who kissed a girl who kissed a man who kissed a girl who kissed a man who maybe... Straight talking about how the infection is acquired, combined with the many examples we have of those exposed to infected people yet who do not acquire the infection, should suffice to reassure their anxiety. However, some persist and one suspects a potential underlying psychoneurosis. AIDS has become the receptacle of people's health anxieties and phobias. Those who used to be worried about cancer are now worried about AIDS. If only they would worry about smoking! The over-anxious people like this need to be called in for more formal counselling. Underlying hypochondriacal trends and psychoneurosis may become apparent. Occasionally one sees schizophrenic delusions presenting as AIDS anxieties.

Sometimes the only way to allay people's fears is by letting them have the antibody test.

THE ANTIBODY TEST

The main way of finding out if a person is infected with the human immuno-deficiency virus is to take a blood sample and test it for antibodies to the virus. The antibodies to the virus are present three months after the infection was contracted. If the test shows up positive this means that the person was exposed to the virus at some stage in their life and we assume that the virus is still present, even if it is latent. If the virus is present the person is infectious and may pass it on by blood or sex. They become reliably present three months after the infection was contracted (except in the case of newborn babies, see pages 64-5).

False negatives can result if the test is done too early. It takes three months from the time of infection for the antibodies to develop, and if a person is tested during this incubation period the antibodies will not show up. It is also possible for tests to show up negative if it is done too late. If a person's immune system is already breaking down, they may lose their antibodies. For this reason it is better for doctors to use their clinical judgement than to rely too heavily on tests.

There are arguments for and against testing. On the face of it, it might seem better if everybody with fears about the virus took a test, so that their minds could be put at rest if the test proves negative. But what if the test proves positive? Does the patient really want to know that they have this potentially lethal infection with all the stigma attached to it? The social consequences, the work consequences, the practical difficulty of getting life assurance or a mortgage, even, sometimes, of getting medical or dental treatment where health-care workers are ill-informed and afraid of infection, as well as the personal consequences in terms of future life expectancy and dealing with one's current sex life have to be faced. And if the test proves negative, the person may then have a false feeling of security and may not take the necessary precautions to keep themselves free of the virus. Counselling must address the problem of people going out to celebrate their negative result and getting infected that night!

Many gay groups have reservations about the test and may actually advise people against having it done. Nobody wants to see the gains made by gay groups in achieving recognition for their cause to be treated equally and without stigma eroded by this epidemic. They have responded in a very positive way by helping people to be informed about altering their lifestyle to prevent spread of infection. They are especially conscious of the considerable psychological and emotional morbidity that occurs when a patient is informed that they are infected. They are in touch with the situation both from personal experience and through counselling services.

It may be argued that people who know they are HIVab+ might be more careful in following safe sex guidelines, but everybody should follow these guidelines anyway, because the other person may be infected. If you are not infected you must take steps to ensure that you do not become infected, and if you are infected you must be sure that you do not pass the infection on. Essentially it comes down to stable, monogamous relationships and safe sex practices, whether you have been tested or not. This means that there is in general no special advantage to having the test, and there may be disadvantages.

People who have had the test and are HIVab+ need special counselling and advice, and where there is a high level of infection in an area, health-care workers may be overworked and not have the time to give to each HIVab+ patient. In areas where the infection rate is low, counselling services may not be available either, as people may simply not have experience of the infection.

On the other hand, for people who are in low-risk groups and who are unlikely to be infected, an antibody test may put them at ease. Testing carried out with consent, counselling and confidentiality serves many purposes. It serves as a marker for those at risk and, with counselling, there is a substantially greater degree of compliance with safe sex practices in those who have been tested. For those about to embark upon a stable relationship, either homosexual or heterosexual, it serves as a marker that they are free from infection and free to have penetrative sex once they follow the three months guideline and remain faithful to each other. In areas of lower prevalence it allows health-caring resources to see the people who are infected and target their resources towards them in an effort to contain the infection. And for people who wish to have children but who feel that they or their partner might be infected, a test is essential, as there is a very high risk of an infected mother passing on the virus to her baby, and indeed pregnancy is itself a co-factor and an infected woman has a 50 per cent chance of progressing to AIDS if she becomes pregnant.

Anyone who is anxious to have an HIV test is presumably in a high-risk group, or has been engaging in high-risk activities, and in this case, whether or not they are HIVab+, they are quite likely to have other sexually transmitted diseases. Because of media interest in AIDS, many people are coming for HIV testing, and fortunately most of them are proving negative, though we are finding many other sexually transmitted diseases, some of them with potentially lethal consequences, such as human papilloma virus infection which causes genital warts, abnormal cervical smears which may express as cancer in years to come. To take an HIVab test without going for a full STD check is to miss a golden opportunity for positive health screening.

If a person wishes to know whether or not they are infected they have a right to know. In Ireland the HIVab test is available at the STD clinics, at the drug unit in Jervis Street Hospital in Dublin, and from GPs. Open and easy access to testing must be maintained, especially to preserve the blood supply free from infection. The last thing that is wanted is for people to donate blood in order to determine their HIV status.

CONSENT, CONFIDENTIALITY AND COUNSELLING

If there is to be testing the basic ground rules of dealing with AIDS must be observed: the three Cs are Consent, Confidentiality and Counselling.

There is no place for testing without consent, and that would be the attitude of those who have experience of dealing with HIV-infected patients and those with AIDS. In those instances where people have been faced with a positive test which has been taken without their consent, there is substantially more psychological and emotional morbidity on hearing the result.

Some people advocate compulsory testing, but these are usually not people involved in the day-to-day realities of dealing with patients. Often they are also those who would find it difficult to seek consent because they are afraid and inhibited to ask about a person's sexuality or history of drug abuse. The one thing about this infection is that it holds up a mirror to society, and we have to face ourselves, warts and all. Before one makes statements about the ethics of testing one has to be able to stand in front of that mirror.

To contain and control an epidemic we need information about its prevalence and spread. Sir Robert Doll, the English epidemiologist, suggested that certain selected groups should be tested anonymously to ascertain the spread of infection. The groups could include antenatal patients, routine samples of blood taken in hospitals, and samples from health-screening sites. This has already been done in some retrospective surveys, on the prevalence of HIV infection in STD clinic attenders and amongst drug abusers. The problem about prospective surveys is what to do with a positive result when you are unable to communicate this information to the patient concerned. This is a real ethical dilemma, as there is no doubt that the information would allow us to target our health-care provision and education programmes to where they are most needed, but if the samples are blinded for identity and consent has not been obtained, one cannot tell a person that they are infected. Perhaps the best approach is one of common sense: why not seek consent in the first place? It is not such a difficult thing to do.

Testing implies an invasion into people's privacy in a very sensitive area, and in Ireland homosexuality remains a criminal offence, which makes confidentiality essential. Those whom we are most anxious to help, counsel and advise regarding HIV infection and STD in general, the core groups, will not come near our clinics or health-care agencies if there is the slightest question of mandatory testing or reporting of infected cases, or breach of confidentiality. When mandatory reporting was introduced in Sweden in the autumn of 1986, attendance at the STD clinics fell by 50 per cent, so 50 per cent were lost to diagnosis, counselling and help. Our policy must be one of consent, complete confidentiality and privacy as regards this test, with attendant counselling.

There is a dilemma when a doctor is faced with a patient whom he or she knows to be infected and raises the question of their partner, either homosexual or heterosexual. However, it must be left entirely to the patient to make the decision to inform the partner. It would be best if they took the action themselves, but if they seek help in doing so the counsellor could be involved. In practice, with good counselling, this has been easy to achieve and once informed, patients have been concerned to ensure that their partner's health was safeguarded.

If and when there is any treatment available for this infection, the argument may swing completely and most people will want to be screened.

SAFE SEX GUIDELINES

Prevention is the only cure. Recognition that the infection can only be contracted by certain routes gives us the greatest weapon to fight its spread. It is quite clear that transmission of the virus is related to penetrative sexual intercourse, either homosexual or heterosexual. There is no evidence of spread from body contact, or even from ingesting potentially contaminated fluids such as sperm, as in oral sex. It is also quite clear that strictures for celibacy are not likely to succeed except for a few individuals. Infections have been around for a long time, the dangers of syphilis, which was just as lethal as AIDS until the advent of penicillin in the late 1940s, did not deter many from taking a chance. The sexual urge is one of life's main forces and it reaches its height in late adolescence and the twenties, especially in men, at a time when many do not have the outlet of a marital or other stable relationship.

The Swedes managed to reduce their high prevalence of gonorrhoea in the 1970s by 40 per cent with a simple and effective public health campaign. It recommended three options: **celibacy,** which they did not think was a practical option, **staying with one partner,** which they felt was the ideal (it should be added that it is also necessary for the partner to stick to you) or **use of a condom,** which is a very effective barrier against infection, and pregnancy, so long as you do use it. It does not work sitting in its box! Safe sex guidelines to protect people against the spread of AIDS are much the same.

Safe sex guidelines were primarily formulated for the homosexual community — where sex is seen often as a means of social contact and exchange — as a method of maintaining one's social outlet and replacing penetrative sex with a different kind of sexual expression, which does not involve the risk of infection. It was soon found that following these guidelines enhanced relationships and the pleasure and enjoyment of sex, rather than detracting from it. The guidelines concentrated the mind on the relationship between people, rather than the repetitive, and sometimes fading, pleasure of the ejaculation. There is much in these guidelines that is appropriate to heterosexual sex as well.

Don't drop your trousers for someone you would not leave your wallet or handbag out for! *At least* know their name and address, and preferably have met some of their friends and family to give you some security of their *bona fides*. It is amazing how careless people can be when it comes to choosing a sex partner, even people who are quite fussy in their day-to-day life.

Some people today are establishing a pattern of questioning to determine the risk status of a potential partner. One enquires what travels they have been on, where they hang out, who their friends are, and eventually, before one takes the jump, what their previous love life has been like. Though this may sound a bit off-putting, many of those I have spoken to tell me that it works 'like a dream' in practice and prospective lovers are much happier that the subject has been raised and addressed, as often they have the same underlying insecurity and were afraid to discuss it. Certainly one should be relaxed if one is to achieve sexual fulfilment. After all, the brain is the most important sexual organ.

For those who are not too sure of their lovers and who wisely wish to play safe, the safe sex guidelines basically counsel against the exchange of body fluids: in other words against any practice whereby one person receives the body fluids (semen, saliva, blood, etc.) into their body.

Completely safe practices would include hugging, holding, cuddling, body rubbing and social dry kissing as well as mutual masturbation.

Possibly risky activities might include french (wet) kissing, oral receptive sex (with the penis) and water sports (urinating on the skin). Oral-genital sex, both with the vagina in the female (cunnilingus) and with the anus (rimming) in the male, is also included. Although these activities are included as possibly risky, it must be emphasised that there are no known case reports of transmission solely related to these practices and that they are thought of as possibly risky on purely theoretical grounds only. For instance we have already mentioned that it would require two or three pints of saliva to transmit sufficient virus to establish an infection.

Risky activities would include swallowing semen, water

sports in the mouth or on broken skin, sharing objects such as dildos or sex-toys or douching. Again they would be theoretically considered risky but no cases relating to these factors alone have been found.

Very risky activities would include anal or vaginal intercourse without a condom and fisting or insertion of the hand into the anus. Particularly receptive anal sex has been shown to be a very efficient means of acquiring the infection.

Condoms can offer considerable protection when they are consistently used. The virus cannot penetrate the latex membranes, and spermicides have some anti-HIV activity when tested in the laboratory. They must be worn throughout intercourse to provide an efficient barrier. They must not break or protection would be lost. Most condoms are designed for vaginal intercourse and are highly reliable in that context if constantly used. Use of a lubricant decreases the chances of breakage. Studies of prostitutes who consistently use condoms in Denmark and Germany have shown a zero rate of infection with HIV and many other sexually transmitted diseases.

However, use of the condom for anal intercourse puts extra strain upon the strength of the membranes, which are often designed to be of the lightest possible consistency to achieve maximum sensitivity. There are some brands available which claim extra strength but it is important to establish that this claim is based on fact rather than reputation and marketing. Plentiful use of lubrication will help protect against breakage. There are some animal skin condoms available made from sheep intestines that are claimed to be much stronger, quite sensitive and natural, but are expensive. However they can be reused.

People do not like using condoms if they can help it. They may interfere with the joy of sex, but so too can an anxiety about the risk of infection. Some people are embarrassed to suggest using a condom as it implies lack of confidence in the potential partner. Many do not know how to use one reliably and when to put it on. Before dinner? After dinner? At the disco? Or on getting home ? The best place is the natural one, when both partners are sufficiently aroused to contemplate sex and happy in their relationship with each other. Use of the condom is a caring act if you or your partner are unsure of your health status. It cares for you and your partner and prevents infection. It should be gently unrolled on the erect penis, taking care not to tear it with rough finger nails. A space should be left at the top for the ejaculate. After intercourse it should be held on withdrawing and then discarded, taking care of the susceptibility of others who might stumble upon it.

Alcohol has a powerful effect upon our inhibitions and judgement. No matter how well conversant we may be on safe sex guidelines, the use of condoms and choice of partners, a few drinks can throw all that to the wind and one may end up infected. So 'stick to your limit' and not just when you're driving!

CHAPTER 6

QUESTIONS AND ANSWERS

with Dr Zachary Johnson

Gay Byrne interviewed Dr John Green, one of Britain's most experienced AIDS counsellors, on RTE Radio 1 on Wednesday 11 March 1987. He conducted a second interview the following morning with Dr Zachary Johnson of the Eastern Health Board. The spread of the human immuno-deficiency virus (HIV) in Ireland, its transmission and general issues relating to AIDS were discussed. The following week one of the producers from the Gay Byrne Show interviewed several young men from the midlands area on the show. It was obvious that there was considerable potential for spread of the HIV amongst the heterosexual community with individuals having multiple sexual partners.

These interviews aroused considerable public interest and many letters and phone calls were received by the Gay Byrne programme on the question of AIDS. General answers to some of these queries were broadcast by Gay Byrne over the next few days on the radio. However, it became obvious that the depth of public concern together with the volume of requests for more information was such that it would be only possible to answer a small number of queries over the radio. People were obviously anxious and we looked at ways of providing them with access to the sort of information they needed. The concept of a confidential phone-in service was suggested and this had a lot of merit as it would enable each caller to be given an individual answer and at the same time it would enable sufficient information about the case to be elicited to make sure the advice was as specific as possible.

The objects of the AIDS helpline were to provide people with information on HIV infection in order to help them to avoid becoming infected, to direct those requiring further counselling, investigation or treatment to the appropriate agencies, to allay unnecessary fears about HIV infection and to identify major areas of public concern about HIV infection as a guide to provision of further services, especially hotline type services.

RTE installed a mini outside broadcast facility in the Telecom building for the duration of the helpline operation. Gay Byrne conducted four live interviews with doctors in the helpline operations room during the Gay Byrne Show. This appeared to cause a massive increase in calls. Further interviews were conducted for RTE Television News, the Today at Five radio programme, and the Morning Ireland radio programme. In addition, reporters from all the main newspapers called in and were briefed on the operation.

In all of these interviews, the mode of transmission of HIV infection was stressed and the lack of risk from casual social contact emphasised. Also, it was pointed out that in the absence of a vaccine or effective therapy, the only effective defence against the spread of HIV infection is information. If everyone acted on the information available at present, the spread of the virus would come rapidly to a halt in Ireland. Thus the opportunity provided by the publicity associated with the AIDS helpline was used to try to get basic information on the virus to as many people as possible through the media.

THE RESULTS

Over 900 calls were received by the AIDS helpline and details of 893 of these were noted and analysed.

It would appear that it was the 'hippie' generation in the main who were reached by the helpline. The average age of women callers was older (thirty-seven years) than that of men (thirty-four years). Unfortunately, there seems to have been less response amongst the young.

No. of Callers	Sex	Marital Status	Age
893	Male 47% Female 53%	Married 70% Single 27% Widowed 3%	Range 12-85 Average 36 Over 3/4 calls from people over 30 2/3 of calls in 20s and 30s. 1.6% under 20

THE QUESTIONS

We give here a summary of the questions asked and of the replies to them given by the helpline counsellors. Where Dr Freedman wishes to expand on these replies, his comments are given as 'Answers' after the helpline comments. What is said in this chapter overlaps considerably with what is said in the rest of the book, and you are directed at times to specific places in the book where you will find more information on topics raised here.

Blood transfusion One caller in ten was concerned about the risks of blood transfusion and 80 per cent of such calls were from women. Considering the simple message being preached by many health professionals of transmission through 'blood and sex', people's anxiety is quite understandable. These callers received reassurance that no cases of HIV infection due to blood transfusion had been documented in this country to date and were told of the extensive safety precautions in operation by Pelican House since October 1985. An occasional call related to a blood transfusion received in Africa quite recently, and clearly these were more worrying.

Answer Since the exclusion of high-risk groups from donating, followed by the introduction of testing of blood donations for HIV antibodies, people who receive blood donations are no longer considered to be at risk. In Africa there are insufficient resources to test all blood and in areas of high HIV prevalence blood transfusions can carry a substantial risk of being infected.

It must be pointed out that *donation of blood carries no risk whatsoever*. There is no conceivable way with the sterile disposable equipment used that the donation of blood could lead to infection in the donor. (See pages 41-2.)

Testing for HIV infection Fifty-one calls (6 per cent of total) enquired about the nature, availability and meaning of the HIVab test. These came in equal proportions from men and women. Counsellors tried to establish the caller's level of risk and if this seemed very low, as was often the case, they were discouraged from having the test done. For higher risk people the implications of the test were outlined, and while people were told where and when they could have it done, they were advised to think very carefully before submitting themselves for testing.

Answer HIV infection is tested for by examining a blood sample for the presence of antibodies to the virus. They are reliably present about three months from the time of infection. Their presence means that the person has been exposed to the virus, and that they are infected with the virus which will probably remain in a persistingly infective stage for life. Being 'antibody positive' does not mean that you have AIDS, it merely means that you have been infected by the virus. The chances of progressing to AIDS or other serious illnesses varies from 2 to 10 per cent per annum and have been discussed.

The test is available from genito-urinary (STD or VD) clinics, drug treatment centres and GPs. It is important that one is counselled before the test is taken and one receives post-test counselling also. (See pages 101-5.)

Prostitutes Five per cent of the calls (forty-seven) related to sex with prostitutes — generally heterosexual sex. Eighty-seven per cent of these calls were from men. There were also a few calls from women worried about their husbands having had sex with prostitutes. The risks of having sex with prostitutes were stressed by the counsellors, particularly if the prostitute was a drug addict or operated in a high-risk area such as Central Africa. These callers were generally advised to attend an STD clinic.

Answer The professional prostitute usually makes her clients use condoms, both to protect her client and herself. Condoms have been shown to be a very effective means of prevention of transmission of this infection, as well as many other infections. In Ireland we have not had any positive infected cases yet from prostitute contact either in Ireland or abroad. It is important to develop contact and ways of working with prostitutes so as to increase their general social awareness and help them to look after themselves.

Acupuncture, tattooing, ear-piercing and beauty treatment
Thirty-four calls enquired about the risk of various non-medical procedures that involve the use of needles that penetrate the skin such as acupuncture and tattooing. Eighty-five per cent of these were from women. Some were worried because when they requested sterilisation of needles they were told that there was no need as the needles did not penetrate the blood stream and therefore could be used on more than one client. Although no case of HIV infection transmitted by this means has been documented as yet, there have certainly been documented cases of hepatitis B infection spread in this way. As the prevalence of HIV infection increases, the risks of using unsterilised needles in this type of setting will also increase. Ideally a fresh disposable needle should be used for each client and callers were advised to request this. However, in establishments where needles were being reused, people were advised to satisfy themselves that adequate sterilisation was being carried out using an effective method such as autoclaving.

Answer No cases of HIV infection have been transmitted in this way to date. These procedures are decorative and unnecessary, and with the risk of hepatitis B infection one would feel that the wise person would get up off the chair and walk out at the sight of needles being reused or inappropriately sterilised. The use of a 'steam cabinet' is not sufficient for sterilisation.

Oral sex Thirty-one enquiries were received about oral sex, 87 per cent of these being from men. While the evidence suggests that the risk associated with oral sex is much lower than with anal sex, callers were generally advised to refrain from this practice if they or their partner were either HIV positive or at high risk.

Answer There are no documented cases of HIV being transmitted by oral sex, even when semen is swallowed. However, because of the theoretical potential of infection, people are advising against this practice.

Other sexually transmitted diseases There were twenty-seven calls related to sexually transmitted diseases other than HIV infection. Half of these were from men and half from women. In general the callers were advised to attend STD clinics.

Answer HIV infection is sexually transmitted, and anybody who is anxious about acquiring AIDS should be screened for all the other sexually transmitted diseases too. The use of the AIDS helpline as a means for finding out about sexually transmitted diseases points to the need for more adequate services for sexually transmitted diseases in the country.

Heterosexual affair — spouse Twenty-four callers requested advice in relation to a spouse's previous or current heterosexual affair. Eighty per cent of these calls were from women worried about their husbands' activities. These situations were very delicate but generally callers were reassured if the affair had not been a recent one and if it had occurred in Ireland. In higher risk situations the role of HIV testing and of safer sexual practices was discussed.

Answer Heterosexual transmission of the HIV does happen, but it is rare, particularly in Ireland, where it is seen mainly in the drug-abusing population. Nevertheless, the possible risk still remains, and this causes a lot of anxiety in many people. If anxiety persists after simple reassurance and some risk exists, it would be wiser to have an HIV antibody test to remove the worry. This is particularly important in pre-marital situations or when one is planning to get pregnant.

Transmission via insects There were twenty-three calls from people worried about the possibility of insect transmission of HIV infection. Insects mentioned included mosquitoes, fleas and horse flies. Although the fear appears entirely reasonable in view of the existence of other viruses which can be transmitted by insects, fortunately for HIV infection it was possible to give people complete reassurance that there was no evidence of infection by insects. It was pointed out that in Africa the highest prevalence of HIV infection is in very young children and those over the age of fifteen. This finding does not support transmission of the virus via insects.

Answer There is no evidence of insect vector transmission, the quantity of blood ingested by the insect is too small to transmit the infection.

Swimming pools There were twenty-two queries about the safety of swimming pools — 73 per cent of these callers were women. Callers were reassured that transmission via this route has not been documented and is very unlikely as the virus is destroyed by chlorine ions. However, the inadvisability of bathing with open wounds or sores and the importance of proper maintenance of swimming pools were stressed.

Answer The HIV is a virus that is transmitted by direct inoculation. There have been no cases reported of people being infected in a swimming pool. Transmission would be impossible unless they have sex in the swimming pool.

Homosexual affairs Nineteen callers were worried about homosexual affairs which they had had. They were counselled on the importance of HIV testing and on safer sexual practices as well as the importance of not donating blood.

Answer Homosexual sex does carry an appreciably higher risk of infection with this virus. It is most strongly associated with receptive anal intercourse. Safer sex practices should be encouraged as well as care in the choice of partner. Antibody testing may be appropriate with counselling and concurrent checking for other sexually transmitted diseases.

Safe sex There were nineteen calls enquiring about safer sexual practices. Twelve of these were from men and seven from women. The risks of anal intercourse, especially receptive anal intercourse, were explained. The efficacy and risks of using condoms were also outlined.

Answer Safe sex practices once consistently observed can be entirely protective against acquiring this infection and provide a valuable means of allowing people to pursue a fulfilling sex life without the risk of infection. Condoms are a most effective barrier for protection and prevention of spread of infection. Their use should be encouraged, particularly where sex partners are not well known to each other or where either partner is at risk. Safe sex practices have been shown to be entirely effective in preventing the spread of infection to date.

Dentistry Eighteen calls enquiring about the risks of dentistry were received. Seventy per cent of these were from men. Although it was pointed out that there is a possibility of transmission through this route, the HIV virus appears to be much less infectious than the hepatitis B virus and standard practices used by dentists to prevent transmission of hepatitis B infection should be adequate to prevent HIV transmission also. However, callers were recommended to check that their dentist carries out adequate sterilisation procedures.

Answer It is noteworthy that in America where 1.5 million people are infected with this virus that there has been no evidence of substantial numbers of people being infected outside the recognised risk groups. This suggests that transmission by such procedures as dentistry is very unlikely. No cases have been documented as having been transmitted in this way.

General medical problems Eighteen callers made enquiries about general medical problems not directly related to HIV infection. The fact that some of the words used in relation to HIV infection, such as immuno-deficiency, also apply to other medical conditions can cause confusion for some people.

Answer The problem is that the signs and symptoms of HIV infection are so non-specific and common that when they are described to any given population, a proportion of those listening will feel that they have them. It is difficult to overcome this problem while also facing the responsibility of informing the public at large.

Transmission of HIV infection via various body fluids There were eighteen calls enquiring about the risk of transmission through various body fluids, such as vomit, blood, urine. Two-thirds of these calls came from women and they were reassured that the virus is not transmitted to non-sexual household contacts of HIVab+ persons. The use of gloves and household bleach for cleaning contaminated areas was recommended.

Answer There has been no evidence of HIV infection through body fluids other than blood and sperm. There was one possible case where the infection could have been transmitted by breast milk. It has been pointed out that although the virus is present in saliva, it would take two to three pints of saliva to have an adequate amount of virus to establish an infection.

Massage parlours There were fifteen enquiries about the risks associated with massage parlours. Not surprisingly, all of these were from men. Clearly the risks in such establishments relate to the type of sexual contact involved and callers were advised accordingly.

Signs and symptoms of AIDS Thirteen people enquired about signs and symptoms of AIDS. Seven of these were male and six female. If the callers appeared to be in a risk group, they were advised to seek medical attention either from their own doctor or from an STD clinic.

Answer The problem about AIDS is that there are no specific signs or symptoms of it and many of the signs or symptoms of HIV infection and AIDS are so non-specific as to be of little use in making a diagnosis. Media and educational campaigns have alerted us to many of these non-specific signs, many of which are found in a normal population and can be the source of considerable anxiety. (See pages 53-62.)

Masturbation Thirteen people enquired whether masturbation carried a risk of HIV infection. Ten of these were male. The means of transmission of the virus was pointed out to all callers and they received reassurance that masturbation does not carry a risk in relation to HIV infection.

Answer Queries about masturbation point out the basic guilt and anxiety felt by many people about sexuality. Obviously transmission cannot occur except if another person is involved, and then it has to be penetrative sexual intercourse. Masturbation is included as one of the safe sex practices.

Intravenous drug abuse Thirteen callers enquired about the risks associated with illicit drug use, 70 per cent of whom were female. Several worried about having had sexual contact with an intravenous drug abuser. Some enquired about the possibility of cleaning needles between users. The extreme dangers associated with the sharing of needles or syringes were emphasised and if appropriate people were referred to drug treatment centres.

Fomites Ten callers enquired about the risks of transmission via fomites, such as cups, plates, door handles, toilet seats, etc. Nine of these calls were from women. The non-transmissibility of HIV infection via this method was emphasised.

Answer Not only would the virus not survive in such hostile environments, but neither would it be able to penetrate the body and establish an infection.

Kissing They were ten calls enquiring about the risks associated with kissing, 60 per cent from women. It was pointed out that although the virus has been isolated from saliva, it is present in such a low concentration that the likelihood of transmission via this means appears to be extremely small.

Answer Studies of households with infected members have shown no evidence of transmission through kissing and even in studies where there was oral-genital contact involving swallowing semen, there were no cases of HIV transmission.

Cranks and hoaxers There were eight calls classified as being crank calls and two hoax calls. Sixty per cent of the cranks were men. In addition, one of the counsellors stated that he had received a further half-dozen hoax or crank type calls, the details of which he did not bother to record. The fact there were so few calls of this nature suggests that the public appears to have taken the AIDS issue very seriously indeed.

Answer It is heartening to see that so few of these calls were received, and in particular the lack of abusive calls is very encouraging and highlights the fact that so many people want more information about this subject.

Artificial insemination There were eight calls enquiring about the risks of artificial insemination, seven from women. It was pointed out that all semen used in this country comes from the British Pregnancy Advice Service and that all donors are carefully screened and tested. Transmission of HIV infection via artificial insemination has been documented in Australia but there have been no cases documented in relation to the Irish suppliers. It was pointed out that the risk associated with artificial insemination appeared to be extremely low, but risk cannot be eliminated altogether.

Answer The practice of storing semen for three months and testing the donors three months after the donation for HIV infection would appear to be a reliable, strong defence against receiving infected semen.

Condoms There were seven calls enquiring about the effectiveness of condoms plus four enquiring about availability. It was pointed out that studies have shown a protective effect against other sexually transmitted diseases by using condoms and also that the incidence of HIV infection appears to be zero among prostitutes who always use condoms. However, the fact that condoms may break occasionally was stressed so that people should not feel that they are totally protected by using condoms. Those requesting information on availability were directed to pharmacies, family planning clinics, etc.

Answer Condoms have been shown to be an extremely reliable and effective means of preventing transmission of HIV as well as other sexually transmitted diseases. Condom breakage in usual sexual practice is quite rare, but when used for anal intercourse they are subjected to stresses and strains for which they were not intended. Lubrication can help prevent tearing.

Living with an HIVab+ person There were seven enquiries about the risks associated with living with an HIVab+ person. The lack of risk associated with casual household contact was stressed. On the other hand, the need for safer sexual practices in situations where the caller was the spouse of an infected person was emphasised, as was the need to avoid pregnancy where either partner was infected.

Answer Living with an HIV-infected person is no problem: it is having sex with them that transmits the virus. There is a large body of evidence that transmission does not occur with ordinary household and social contact.

Stable heterosexual relationships There were six calls from women who appeared to be in stable heterosexual relationships but who were worried about the risk of infection. There appeared to be no other risk factors and all were reassured. However, calls of this nature emphasised the need for a proper information campaign for the public.

Rape There were five calls on the question of rape, four of them from women. In general, these callers were reassured if the incident was not recent and if it occurred in a low-risk geographical area. Alternatively, they were directed to appropriate counselling or treatment facilities.

Answer Rape, involving penetrating sex, carries an unknown potential risk of infection. Fortunately the prevalence of infection in Ireland at present is quite low so one would have to be very unlucky indeed to become infected. If there is any appreciable anxiety, it would be wisest to carry out an HIV antibody test.

Offers of help for AIDS cases Five people, all female, offered their services to help victims of HIV infection. It was an encouraging sign, and undoubtedly there will be a considerable need for voluntary service in caring for AIDS cases in times to come.

Holy communion Four callers enquired about the risks of HIV transmission via holy communion. All were reassured.

Enquiries relating to a media campaign for AIDS Four people wondered if and when a media campaign on AIDS is going to begin. They were told that while the helpline counsellors were fully aware of the need for such a campaign they were not privy to its contents or its scheduled starting date. [This campaign has now started.]

Sterilisation and disinfection Four callers enquired about sterilisation and disinfection of household items and contaminated surfaces. They were reassured that the HIV is relatively fragile and that household bleach is a very effective substance for killing the virus.

Children finding used condoms There were four calls from mothers whose children had found and played with used condoms. It appears that certain places such as school-yards are frequented by courting couples and children occasionally find and play with used condoms in these areas. It was pointed out that, although it is certainly not desirable for children to play with such items, the risk of transmission of HIV infection by this means is virtually non-existent.

Answer There have been no cases documented to be transmitted in this way. To transmit the virus the sperm would have to gain entry into the body, and this would be extremely unlikely to happen.

Calls from HIVab+ persons There were four calls from people who were aware that they were HIVab+. Appropriate counselling was given and people were directed to the relevant support services if they were not already in contact with these.

Answer HIV-infected people require a lot of support and counselling. It would be interesting to know why these people were calling the AIDS helpline rather than being under medical care themselves. The lack of follow-up of HIVab+ persons does not allow counselling for the control or spread of this infection through safe sex practices, which is essential for containment.

Blood donation There were four people enquiring about the risks of HIV infection from donating blood. All were reassured that donating blood carries no risk whatsoever and that disposable needles are used in every case.

Answer It is extremely surprising for most professionals that people could feel that donating blood carries a risk. Many have been reassured and hopefully they will return to their routine donations.

Surgery There were two enquiries about the risks associated with surgery and appropriate reassurance was given.

Answer No cases have been reported of infection being contracted at surgery, even when the surgeon was infected.

Once standard appropriate measures are taken to protect against infection, there should be no risk to a patient.

Sanitary towels There were two enquiries about the risk of HIV infection from sanitary towels. Callers were reassured and appropriate hygiene measures were stressed.

Answer People are concerned about the presence of blood and overlook the basic fact that the infection has to be actually transmitted from one person to another.

Adoption There were three enquiries about the risks of an adopted child being infected. Generally reassurance could be offered because of the age of the children. However, this area is likely to give rise to difficulty as more HIVab+ children are born.

Answer Children who are antibody negative at birth are extremely unlikely to have this infection. Those born antibody positive may have to wait some months until maternal antibodies are cleared to see if the child is infected. (See pages 64-5.) This makes early adoption more difficult which is to the detriment of the child.

Bisexuality There were two calls from women whose husbands had had homosexual affairs and there were two calls from women who had had affairs with bisexual men. The risks were explained to these callers and appropriate referrals made. Clearly, situations like these are one means by which the HIV infection can spread from the high-risk groups to the heterosexual population.

Answer This is an obvious potential risk and points to the necessity of knowing your partner. And just knowing your partner may not be enough — you need to be sure about their activities with people other than yourself. Many married bisexuals conceal their homosexual activity from their wives. But of course bisexuals are not necessarily infected. On the other hand it would seem to be wiser for bisexual men to check their antibody status frequently to ensure that they are not infecting female partners with the potential for a further generation to be infected.

Lesbian transmission Two people were worried about the possibility of transmission between lesbians. While the risk would appear to be very low, it is conceivable that it could occur.

Answer Sexually transmitted disease with lesbian sex is very rare indeed. It basically relates to the lack of penetrative sexual activity. The penis is designed as a transmitting mechanism: it transmits genetic material in the sperm from one person to another.

Enquiries about marriage and pregnancy There were two enquiries from people who had been at some risk of infection and were contemplating marriage and/or pregnancy. The value of HIV testing in this situation was pointed out, and its availability was indicated.

Answer The consequences of the HIV-infected person becoming pregnant are immense, both for themselves and the newborn. If either the mother or the father has any risk of harbouring this infection, they should strongly think about being tested before a child is conceived.

Needle-stick injuries Two people enquired about the risk of needle-stick injury in health-care settings. Although the risks are very low, transmission via this means has been documented and extreme care should be exercised by health-care workers to avoid such injuries.

Answer What is striking is that so few cases of infection have been documented as a result of needle-stick injury, despite the thousands of such injuries that are being followed up both in America and England. (See page 41.)

Enquiries from relatives of HIVab+ cases There were two queries from relatives of individuals who were HIVab+ but not living under the same roof. Appropriate reassurance and counselling were given.

Monogamous homosexual relationships There was an enquiry about the risks associated with monogamous homosexual relations between men. It was pointed out that there was no risk of HIV infection in this situation provided both partners were indeed faithful and provided neither abused illicit drugs.

Answer There is no risk of infection provided you stick to your partner and your partner sticks to you. Some people have an HIVab test before commencing a stable relationship. It must be remembered that it is only valid for the time up to three months before the test, and you should have the test again in another three months to make sure you have not developed antibodies in the meantime. In the three-month hiatus between the two tests, you should follow safe sex guidelines.

Fears in relation to overseas experiences Ninety-three of the callers were worried about some experience they had had overseas, whether this was a heterosexual or homosexual affair or a blood transfusion. Forty-seven callers were concerned about a heterosexual affair that they themselves had had. In thirteen cases the affair had occurred in continental Europe, ten in North America, nine had occurred in the UK and there were seven cases from Africa. There were a further ten calls from people worried about contact with prostitutes overseas, the majority of these having occurred either in continental Europe or the UK. There were eight calls from people whose spouse had had a heterosexual affair overseas, again usually in Europe or North America. There were four calls from people who had had homosexual experiences overseas.

Answer There are pools of high prevalence of this infection building up. It is obvious that even an occasional exposure to these pools could result in a substantial chance of acquiring the infection. In particular one lacks local knowledge overseas and this may make it more difficult to avoid the drug abuser or 'gifted amateur'. People who have had exposures in Africa should be considered to be at special risk.

Sexual orientation of callers In some cases callers stated their sexual preferences and this was noted. Forty-two people stated that they were gay men (5 per cent of all callers). Seventeen were bisexual. It is interesting to note that the helpline was used most by the general public and those least at risk.

CONCLUSION

The enormous public response to the AIDS helpline far exceeded the expectations of the organisers. The size of the reaction suggests that there is a great public concern in relation to AIDS. This may be less surprising when one considers the amount of media coverage given to AIDS in recent times, and in particular the scale of the media campaign mounted in the UK. Clearly, this campaign is likely to have reached the vast majority of people in Ireland as multi-channel TV is available to 75 per cent of the population.

Most callers appeared to be at low risk because the incidents about which they were worried had occurred at a time when the prevalence of HIV infection was probably zero or very low in many parts of the western world. We were concerned that few teenagers or people in their early twenties contacted our service. These are the groups who are probably most at risk at the moment. It was also notable that nearly all calls came from private phones rather than pay-phones, again suggesting that we were not reaching the younger and less well off people.

It was also clear that very few people in the highest risk group in Ireland, namely intravenous drug abusers, contacted the helpline. While this is not surprising it does suggest the need for a special educational programme for this group, rather than relying on traditional media or freephone type approaches.

WHERE TO GO FOR HELP AND ADVICE

STD Clinics
(First-time attenders are requested to arrive early)

St James's Hospital
Genito-Urinary Department
Hospital 7 (Rialto entrance)
St James's Street
Dublin 8
Tel: 01-535245 (direct line)
   Clinics: male and female, Monday-Friday, 4.30-6.00 pm; Dr Fiona Mulcahy, Dr Derek Freedman, Dr Máire Nestor-Nic Ghearailt

Mater Misericordiae Hospital
Out-Patients Department
Eccles Street
Dublin 7
Tel: 01-304488
   Clinics: male, Wednesday and Thursday, 5.00-7.00 pm, female, Tuesday, 4.00-7.00 pm, Thursday, 3.00-4.00 pm; Dr Owen Carey, Dr John Delap, Dr Gerry Bury

Victoria Hospital
Out-Patients Department
Infirmary Road
Cork
Tel: 021-966844

Clinics: Monday, 5.30-7.30 pm, Wednesday, 10.00 am-12 noon, Friday, 2.30-3.00 pm (for advice and information only, by phone); Dr Jack Cantillon, Dr Elizabeth O'Connell

Regional Hospital
Out-Patients Department
Dooradoyle
Limerick
Tel: 061-28111
   Clinics: Friday, 2.30-4.30 pm; Dr Catherine O'Connor

Galway
Tel: 091-64000 (confidential line)
   Clinics: Monday-Friday, 10.00 am-4.00 pm (by appointment only); Dr Emer McHale, Dr Greg Little

Royal Victoria Hospital
Genito-Urinary Medicine Department
Grosvenor Road
Belfast 12
Tel: 084- or 0232-320159
   Clinics: Monday-Friday, 9.00-11.00 am, Monday, Wednesday, Friday, 2.00-3.00 pm; Dr Tom Horner, Dr Raymond Maw, Dr Wallace Dinsmore

Altnagelvin Area Hospital
Glenshane Road
Derry
Tel: 080504- or 0504-45171
   Clinics: Monday, Tuesday, Wednesday, Friday, 9.30-10.30 am; Dr Wallace Dinsmore

Coleraine Hospital
28a Mountsandel Road
Coleraine
Tel: 080265- or 0265-4177
   Clinics: Tuesday, 5.30-6.00 pm (registering time), Friday, 2.00-2.30 pm (registering time); Dr Wallace Dinsmore

National Drugs Advisory and Treatment Centre

Jervis Street Hospital
Jervis Street
Dublin 1
Tel: 01-749358

Clinics: Monday-Friday, 9.30 am-12.30 pm, 2.30-5.30 pm, Saturday, 10.00 am-12.30 pm; Dr Michael Kelly, Dr John O'Connor

National Haemophilia Treatment Centre

Hospital 1
St James's Hospital
St James's Street
Dublin 8
Tel: 01-537941, ext. 2271
Ms Deirdre Flynn, Ms Maeve Foreman

Useful addresses and telephone numbers in Ireland:

Cairde
PO Box 1884
Dublin 1
Tel: 01-307888

AIDS helpline: Tel: 01-307888, Monday, 7.00-10.00 pm, Saturday, 3.00-6.00 pm

Modelled on the Terence Higgins Trust, open to any class, colour, creed or sexual preference. A befriending service for victims of (full blown) AIDS. A volunteer member of Cairde befriends victim, acting as nurse/helper in the victim's own home.

Gay Health Action (GHA)
PO Box 1890
Dublin 1
Tel: 01-710895, Monday-Friday, 11.00 am-4.00 pm

Rape Crisis Centre
70 Lower Lesson Street
Dublin 2
Tel: 01-614911 (24-hour emergency phone service)
   Open: Monday-Friday, 9.30 am-5.30 pm (by appointment only)

Tel-a-Friend
Dublin
Tel: 01-710608
   Sunday-Friday, 8.00-10.00 pm, Saturday, 3.30-6.00 pm, lesbian line, Thursday, 8.00-10.00 pm

Gay Health Action (GHA)
PO Box 87
Cork
Tel: 021-317026, Monday and Friday, 2.00-5.00 pm

AIDS Helpline
PO Box 44
Belfast BT1 1SH
Tel: 084- or 0232-226117, Monday and Friday, 7.30-10.00 pm

Carafriend
Belfast, Tel: 084- or 0232-222023, Monday-Wednesday, 7.30-10.00 pm

Irish Haemophilia Society
29 Eaton Square
Monkstown
County Dublin
Tel: 01-841792

c/o Mrs Joan O'Brien
36 Desmond Square
Cork
Tel: 021-963519

c/o Mrs Nellie Ivess
Bansha
Askeaton
County Limerick
Tel: 061-392412

Counselling for haemophiliacs and their families on all haemophilia-related subjects

Useful addresses and telephone numbers outside Ireland:

The Terence Higgins Trust
BM AIDS
London WC1N 3XX
Tel: Helpline 031- or 01-242-1010, Monday-Friday, 7.00-10.00 pm, Saturday-Sunday, 3.00-10.00 pm

Body Positive
BM AIDS
London WC1N 3XX

A support organisation for those who are HTLV-III sero-positive

London Gay Switchboard
Tel: 031- or 01-837-7324 (24 hours, daily)

GLOSSARY

acquired immune deficiency syndrome: see AIDS

AIDS: The final stage of HIV infection. The sick person's immune system is damaged and the person falls victim to one or more of several opportunistic infections or tumours, and eventually dies. (See pages 53-62.)

AIDS related complex: see ARC

anal intercourse: A form of sexual intercourse in which the penis is inserted into the other person's anus. The person who is inserting their penis is said to be practising 'insertive anal intercourse' and the person receiving the penis is said to be practising 'receptive or passive anal intercourse'. This is a highly risky activity but receptive anal intercourse is more risky than insertive. (This practice is not necessarily confined to homosexuals.)

antibody: A substance produced by the body in response to infection in an attempt to kill off the invader

antibody positive: see HIVab+

antibody test: see HIV antibody test

antigens: Foreign particles, usually proteins, to which the body reacts by producing antibodies

anus: Opening of back passage

ARC (AIDS related complex): Sometimes called 'pre-AIDS', this is a condition that develops in some HIV-infected people. If an HIV-infected person develops certain signs, symptoms or findings over a period of time, but does not have one of the opportunistic infections or tumours characteristic of AIDS, then the diagnosis is ARC. The patient may go on to full AIDS or may recover. (See pages 47-8.)

asymptomatic carrier: A person infected with the HIV but who shows no signs or symptoms. Because they have no symptoms a person may be a carrier without knowing it and may unwittingly pass on the infection to others.

B cells (B lymphocytes): White blood cells, part of the immune system, which produce antibodies

biopsy: A process whereby a piece of body tissue is removed for microscopic examination

bisexual: A person who is attracted to people of both sexes

blood transfusion: Replenishment of a person's blood supply by giving them donated blood

condom: A rubber sheath that fits over the penis during intercourse and collects the semen. Condoms are a good protection against sexually transmitted diseases, including HIV infection.

candidiasis: Infection with the yeast *Candida albicans,* commonly known as 'thrush'

cervix: Neck of the womb

co-factor: Agent that may act along with the main factor in inducing a change. In HIV infection it may induce expression or progression of the illness. In other words it 'triggers off' illness in HIV-infected people.

dementia: Loss of intellectual function, with inability to care for oneself

diagnosis: The process of finding or identifying the nature of a disease

dormant: A virus is said to be 'dormant' if it lies inactive in the body, not reproducing or spreading.

eczema: Inflammatory skin condition

encephalitis: Inflammation of the brain

encephalopathy: Degenerative disease of the brain

exchange of body fluids: Any practice whereby one person receives the body fluids (semen, saliva, etc.) of another into their body. No exchange of body fluids is recommended in the safe sex guideline.

Factor VIII: A concentrate of the clotting factor in blood derived from the pool of many thousands of donors and used to treat haemophiliacs

florid: Showy

foetus: Unborn baby

folliculitis: Inflammation of the hair follicles on the skin of the body

gastrointestinal tract: The whole digestive system from mouth to anus

gay: Homosexual, particularly of men

genitals (genitalia): Sexual organs. External parts of the reproductive system of the male or female.

genome: The complete genetic information which describes an organism

haemophiliac: Person suffering from a blood clotting factor deficiency. The blood of haemophiliacs doesn't clot properly. The reason haemophiliacs were a risk group is that many of them received blood products made from the blood of donors who were infected. All blood donations are now tested and it is very unlikely that haemophiliacs will be infected in the future.

herpes: Inflammation of the skin caused by infection with herpes virus. Characterised by collections of small blisters which break down into ulcers. There are many types of herpes and the most well known, perhaps, is *Herpes simplex* which usually causes lesions around the mouth and/or the genitals and is sexually transmissible.

heterosexual: A person who is attracted to people of the opposite sex

high-risk groups: Groups of people who have been at high risk of becoming infected: haemophiliacs, homosexuals, drug abusers and their babies

HIV (human immuno-deficiency virus): The virus that causes AIDS and milder related conditions

HIVab: The HIV antibody

HIVab+: HIV antibody positive. A person who is tested for HIV antibody and whose test proves positive. This means they are carrying the virus whether they have symptoms or not. It does not mean that they have AIDS, but they may progress to AIDS with time.

HIV antibody test: The test for antibodies to the HIV. It is difficult to test people for the virus itself but the antibody test is readily available. The antibodies to the virus form several weeks after infection and are reliably present after three months.

HIV infection: Having the virus. An HIV-infected person is not necessarily ill, but they have the potential to eventually progress to AIDS.

homosexual: A person who is attracted to people of the same sex

host: A person infected with a virus or other parasite

HTLV-III: Human T cell lymphotropic virus, type III, now known as HIV

immune system: The body's system of defence against infection

immuno-compromise/immuno-deficiency/immuno-deficit/immuno-depression/immuno-suppression: Damage to the immune system

inoculation: Impregnation of the body with a foreign substance

insect vector: Insect carrier

intravenous drug abuse: Injecting illegal addictive drugs such as heroin into a vein with a needle

Kaposi's sarcoma: A type of cancer particularly associated with AIDS

latent: A virus is said to be 'latent' if it lies inactive in the body.

lesbian: Homosexual woman

lesion: Visible damage, particularly on the skin, such as lump, wart, node

libido: Sex drive

low-risk groups: People apparently at low risk of infection; not haemophiliacs, homosexuals or intravenous drug abusers

lymph glands: Collection of lymphoid tissue at various locations in the body. They serve as a defence by removing poisons or foreign particles from the lymphotic fluid. They are the main source of lymphocytes of the blood and play a role in antibody formation.

lymphoma: Cancer of the lymphoid tissue

meningitis: Inflammation of the membranes of the brain and spinal cord

needle-stick injury: Injury to health-care workers by pricking themselves with a needle. Health-care workers may be worried if the needle has been used on an HIV-infected person but the risk is practically nil.

nitrites: Drugs taken to produce a 'high' particularly in sexual intercourse. This is common among homosexuals.

node: Small tumour
nodule: Small node

opportunistic infection: Infections that nab the opportunity to attack a person whose defence system is damaged. It is from these infections or from opportunistic tumours that AIDS patients usually die. These infections would not normally cause disease in a healthy person.
oral sex/oral genital sex: Insertion of the penis into another person's mouth or the tongue into another person's vagina or anus. Where one person receives the other person's penis into the mouth and particularly if semen is swallowed, this is known as oral receptive sex.
orgasm: Peak of sexual excitement

paediatric: To do with children
palate: Roof of the mouth
penetrative: Involving penetration of the body (usually the insertion of the penis into the vagina in heterosexual intercourse, and into the anus with homosexual intercourse)
peri-anal: Around the anus
peri-oral: Around the mouth
persistent generalised lymphadenopathy (PGL): Persistent, generalised swelling of the lymph glands, particularly associated with HIV infection. (See pages 46-7.)
PGL: see persistent generalised lymphadenopathy
***Pneumocystis carinii* pneumonia:** A type of pneumonia particularly associated with AIDS
poppers: see nitrites
presentation: The symptoms or illness with which a person comes to the doctor
prognosis: The outlook or probable outcome of a disease
provirus: The genetic information of a virus that is integrated into the host cell

rectum: Back passage
replication: Process of duplicating or reproducing. As applied to genes and DNA, it is the process by which DNA makes copies of itself when a cell divides, or when new viruses are formed.
retina: Back of the eyeball
retinitis: Inflammation of the back of the eyeball

saliva: Spittle

semen: Fluid ejaculated by a man at orgasm

sero-conversion illness: A flu-like illness that occurs in some HIV-infected people at around the time the antibodies are being formed. It often goes undiagnosed.

sexually transmitted diseases (STD): Infections which can be spread by sexual intercourse

signs: Visible manifestations of disease

silent infection or tumour: One that has no signs or symptoms

STD clinic: Clinic where sexually transmitted diseases are treated (genito-urinary medical clinic)

symptoms: Complaints or subjective indicators of a disease or disorder noticed by the patients themselves

syndrome: Combination of signs and/or symptoms that form a distinct clinical picture indicative of a particular disorder

syphilis: A sexually transmitted disease

systemic drug: Drug that affects the whole system

T cells (T lymphocytes): White blood cells that are part of the immune system

T4 lymphocytes (T4 cells): Particular group of T cells that act as master regulators of the immune system. When activated they may initiate antibody production and cytotoxic killer cell activity.

T8 lymphocytes (T8 cells): Group of T cells that function to suppress the immune response and also act as cytotoxic or killer cells against foreign agents

thrush: A yeast infection in the mouth or vagina, normally irritative but harmless. It may become a serious problem in AIDS patients.

transfusion recipients: People who receive blood transfusions

transmission: Passing on of the virus

tumour: Cancerous or non-cancerous growth

virus: Tiny infectious agent, capable of replication, but only within living host cells.

BIBLIOGRAPHY

Books

British Medical Association, *AIDS and You. An Illustrated Guide,* 1987

Gay Health Action, *AIDS Information Booklet,* 1986

Gottlieb, Michael et al., *Current Topics in AIDS,* John Wiley, 1987 (in press)

Green, John and David Miller, *AIDS — The Story of a Disease,* Grafton Books, 1986

Institute for the Advanced Study of Human Sexuality, *Safe Sex in the Age of Aids,* Citadel Press, Secaucus, New Jersey, 1986

Institute of Medicine, National Academy of Sciences, *Mobilizing Against AIDS — The Unfinished Story of a Virus,* Harvard Univeristy Press, 1986

Miller, David, Jonathan Weber and John Green (eds), *The Management of AIDS Patients,* Macmillan, 1986

Weber, Jonathan and Annabel Ferriman, *AIDS Concerns You,* Pagoda Books, 1986

General and epidemiological papers

Curran, James. W. et al., 'The epidemiology of AIDS. Current status and future prospects', *Science,* vol. 229 (1985), pp. 1352-7

Freedman, Derek, 'AIDS — the uncertain future', *Irish Medical Journal,* vol. 80 (1987), pp. 77-8

International Conference on Acquired Immuno-Deficiency Syndrome, 14-17 April 1985, Atlanta, Georgia, selected papers, *Annals of Internal Medicine,* vol. 103 (1985), pp 653-781

Melbye, Mads, 'The natural history of human T lymphotropic virus-III infection: the cause of AIDS', *British Medical Journal,* vol. 292 (1986), pp. 5-11

Moss, A.R., 'AIDS and intravenous drug use: the real heterosexual epidemic', *British Medical Journal,* vol. 294 (1987), pp. 389-90

Polk, B.F., R. Fox and R. Brookmeyer, 'Predictions of the Acquired Immune Deficiency Syndrome developing in a cohort of seropositive homosexual men', *New England Journal of Medicine,* no. 316 (1987), pp. 61-6

Sunday World, 'Survey on knowledge of AIDS in Ireland', 8 February 1987

United States Public Health Service, *Surgeon General's Report on Acquired Immune Deficiency Syndrome,* Washington, November 1986. Also published in *Irish Medical Journal,* vol. 80 (1987), p. 81

Papers relating to the virus

Gallo, Robert, 'The first human retrovirus', *Scientific American,* December 1986, pp. 78-88

Gallo, Robert, 'The AIDS virus', *Scientific American,* January 1987, pp. 39-48

Kingsley, L.A. et al., 'Risk factors for seroconversion to human immuno-deficiency virus among male homosexuals (results from the Multicentre AIDS Cohort Study)', *The Lancet,* no. 8529 (1987), pp. 345-8

Popovic, Mikulas et al., 'Detection, isolation and continuous production of cytopathic retovirus (HTLV-III) from patients with AIDS and pre-AIDS', *Science,* vol. 224 (1984), pp. 497-500

Schüpbach, Jörg et al., 'Frequent detection and isolation of cytopathic retroviruses (HTLV-III) from patients with AIDS and at risk for AIDS', *Science,* vol. 224 (1984), pp. 500-05.

Wong-Staal, Flossie and Robert Gallo, 'Human T-lymphotropic retroviruses', *Nature,* vol. 317 (1985), pp. 395-403